Keto Air Fryer Diet Cookbook

Tasty and Delicious Vegetables Recipes to Effortless your Health

River Hunt

Table of Contents:

Baked Lamb Chops

Preparation Time:

10 minutes

Cooking Time:

20 minutes

Serve: 5

Ingredients:

5 lamb rib chops
1 garlic clove, grated
2 tbsp olive oil
1 tsp paprika
1/2 tsp smoked paprika
1 tsp cumin
1/2 tbsp oregano

Directions:

1.In a small bowl, mix together paprika, smoked paprika, cumin, oregano, garlic, and 1 tbsp olive oil.

2.Coat lamb chops with spice mixture and place in the refrigerator for 3 hours. Heat remaining 1 tbsp olive oil in a pan over medium-high heat. Once the oil is hot then place lamb chops and cook for 3 minutes or until browned.

3.Select Bake mode. Set time to 16 minutes and temperature 375 F then press START. The air fryer display will prompt you to ADD FOOD once the temperature is reached then place lamb chops in the air fryer basket.

4.Turn lamb chops halfway through. Serve and enjoy.

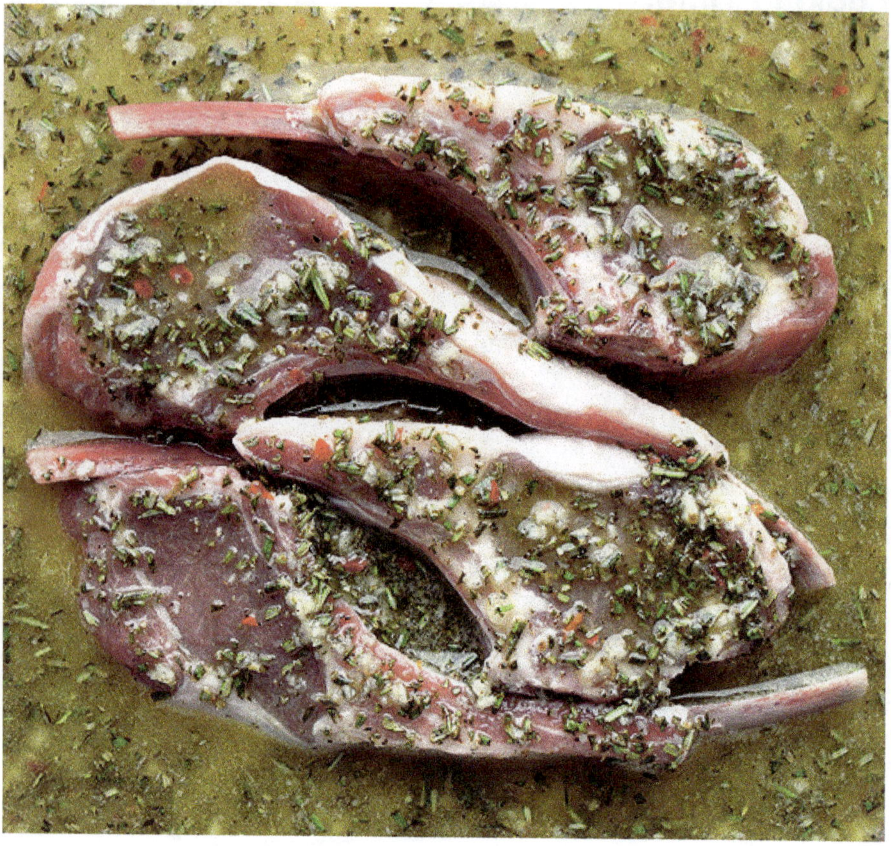

Lemon Garlic Sirloin Steak

Preparation Time:

10 minutes

Cooking Time:

30 minutes

Serve: 6

Ingredients:

2 lbs sirloin steak, cut into
1-inch pieces
2 garlic cloves, minced
1 1/2 cups fresh parsley, chopped
1/2 tsp black pepper
3 tbsp fresh lemon juice
1 tsp dried oregano
1/4 cup water
1/4 cup olive oil
1 tsp salt

Directions:

1.Add all ingredients except beef into the large bowl and mix well together. Pour bowl mixture into the large zip-lock bag.

2.Add beef into the bag and shake well and refrigerate for 1 hour. Select Bake mode.

3.Set time to 30 minutes and temperature 400 F then press START. The air fryer display will prompt you to ADD FOOD once the temperature is reached then place marinated beef in the air fryer basket. Serve and enjoy.

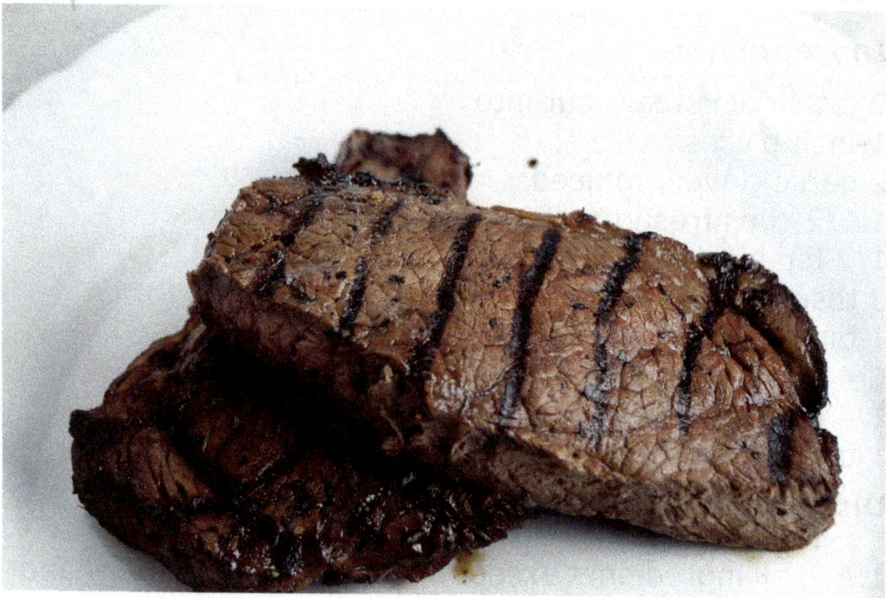

Flavorful Air Fryer Kabab

Preparation Time:

10 minutes

Cooking Time:

10 minutes

Serve: 4

Ingredients:

1/2 lb ground beef
1/2 lb ground pork
4 garlic cloves, minced
1/2 tsp onion powder
1 tsp chili powder
1/4 tsp paprika
1/4 cup fresh parsley, chopped
1 tbsp olive oil
1 tsp salt

Directions:

1.Add all ingredients into the mixing bowl and mix until well combined.

2.Place in refrigerator for 30 minutes. Divide mixture into the 4 portions and make sausage shape kabab. Select Air Fry mode.

3.Set time to 10 minutes and temperature 375 F then press START.

4.The air fryer display will prompt you to ADD FOOD once the temperature is reached then place kabab in the air fryer basket. Turn kabab halfway through. Serve and enjoy

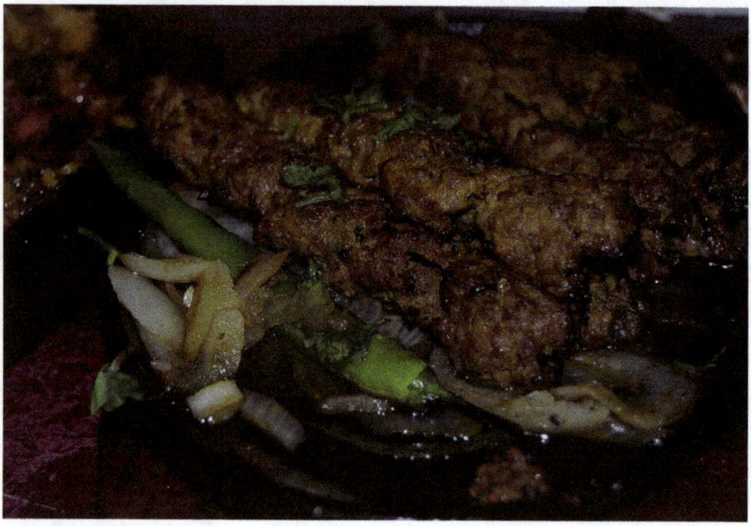

Baked Lamb Patties

Preparation Time:

10 minutes

Cooking Time:

15 minutes

Serve: 4

Ingredients:

1 lb ground lamb
1 tsp chili pepper
½ tsp ground allspice
1 tsp ground cumin
1/4 cup fresh parsley, chopped
1/4 cup onion, minced
1 tbsp ginger garlic paste
1/4 tsp pepper
1 tsp kosher salt

Directions:

1.Add all ingredients into the large bowl and mix until well combined. Make four equal shapes of patties from meat mixture.

2.Select Bake mode. Set time to 15 minutes and temperature 400 F then press START.

3.The air fryer display will prompt you to ADD FOOD once the temperature is reached then place patties in the air fryer basket.

4.Turn patties after 8 minutes. Serve and enjoy.

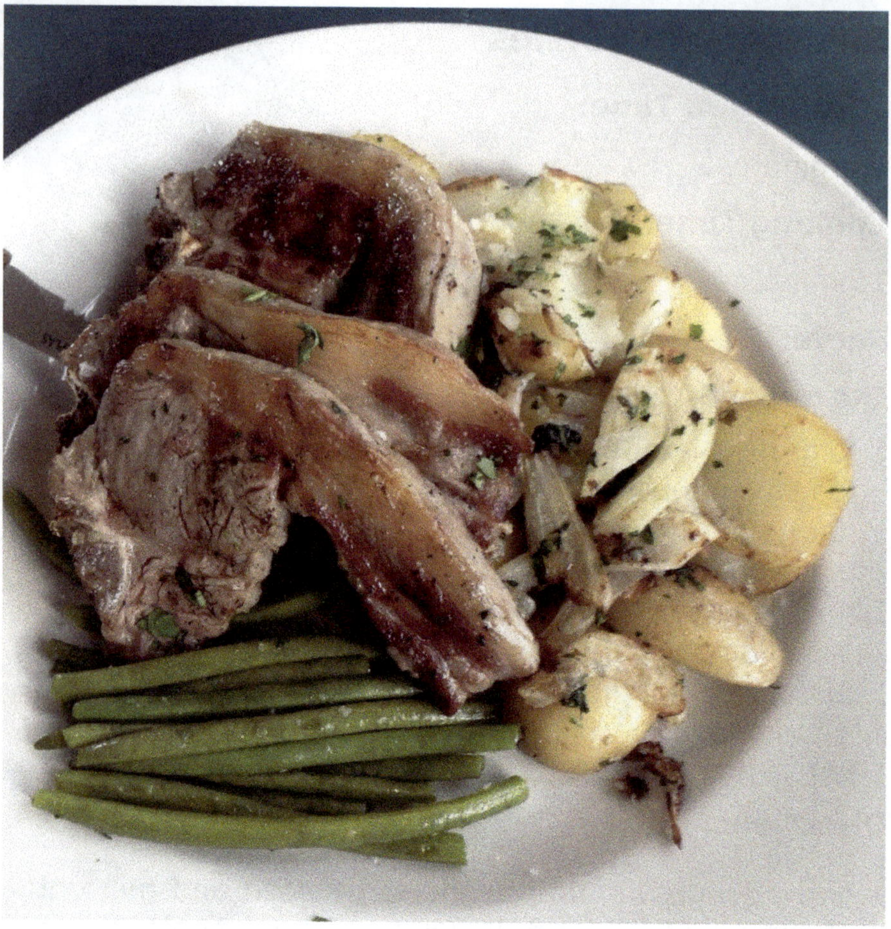

Greek Beef Casserole

Preparation Time:

10 minutes

Cooking Time:

1 hour 30 minutes

Serve: 6

Ingredients:

1 lb lean stew beef, cut into chunks
4 oz black olives, sliced
7 oz can tomatos, chopped
1 tbsp tomato puree
2 cups beef stock
2 tbsp olive oil
1/4 tsp garlic powder
2 tsp herb de Provence
3 tsp paprika

Directions:

1.Heat oil in a pan over medium heat. Add meat to the pan and cook until browned.

2.Add stock, olives, tomatoes, tomato puree, garlic powder, herb de Provence, and paprika. Stir well and bring to boil.

3.Transfer meat mixture into the baking dish. Cover dish with foil. Select Bake mode.

4.Set time to 60 minutes and temperature 350 F then press START.

5.The air fryer display will prompt you to ADD FOOD once the temperature is reached then place the baking dish in the air fryer basket. Stir well and cook for 30 minutes more. Serve and enjoy.

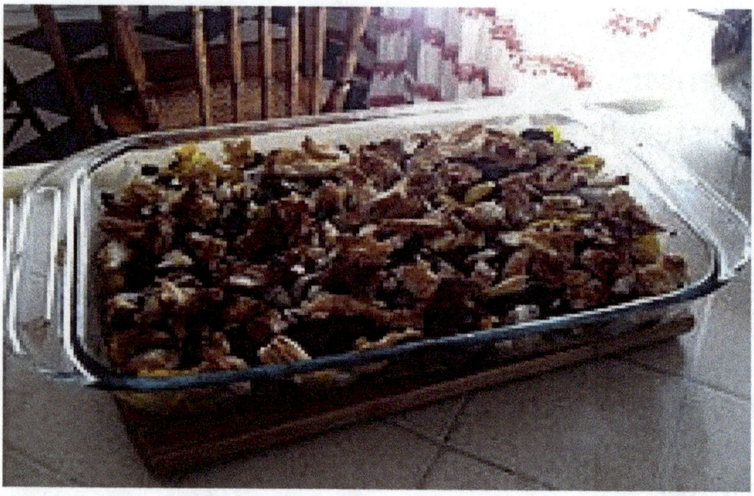

Mini Meatloaf

Preparation Time:

10 minutes

Cooking Time:

25 minutes

Serve: 2

Ingredients:

1/2 lb ground beef
1 1/2 tbsp almond flour
1 egg, lightly beaten
2 olives, chopped
1 tbsp green onion, chopped
1/2 small onion, chopped
1 tbsp chorizo, chopped
Pepper Salt

Directions:

1.In a large bowl, mix together all ingredients until well combined. Transfer meat mixture into the small baking dish. Cover dish with foil.

2.Select Bake mode. Set time to 25 minutes and temperature 400 F then press START.

3.The air fryer display will prompt you to ADD FOOD once the temperature is reached then place the baking dish in the air fryer basket. Serve and enjoy.

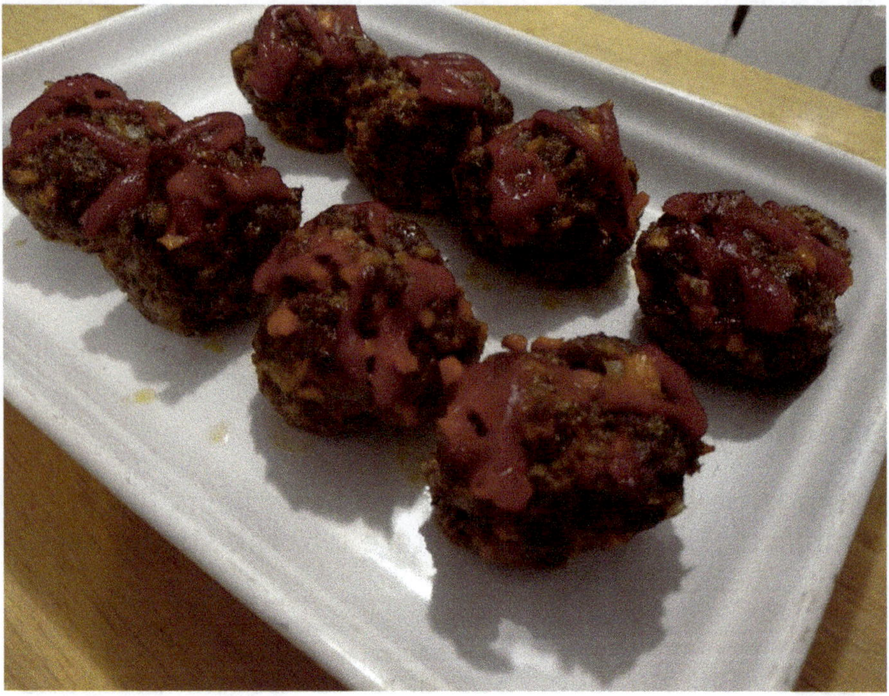

Flavorful Beef Satay

Preparation Time:

10 minutes

Cooking Time:

8 minutes

Serve: 2

Ingredients:

1 lb beef flank steak, sliced into long strips
1 tbsp fish sauce
2 tbsp olive oil
1 tsp hot sauce
1 tbsp Swerve
1 tbsp ginger garlic paste
1 tbsp soy sauce
1/2 cup parsley, chopped
1 tsp ground coriander

Directions:

1.Add all ingredients into the zip-lock bag and shake well.

2.Place into the refrigerator for 1 hour. Select Air Fry mode. Set time to 8 minutes and temperature 400 F then press START.

3.The air fryer display will prompt you to ADD FOOD once the temperature is reached then place marinated meat in the air fryer basket. Stir halfway through. Serve and enjoy.

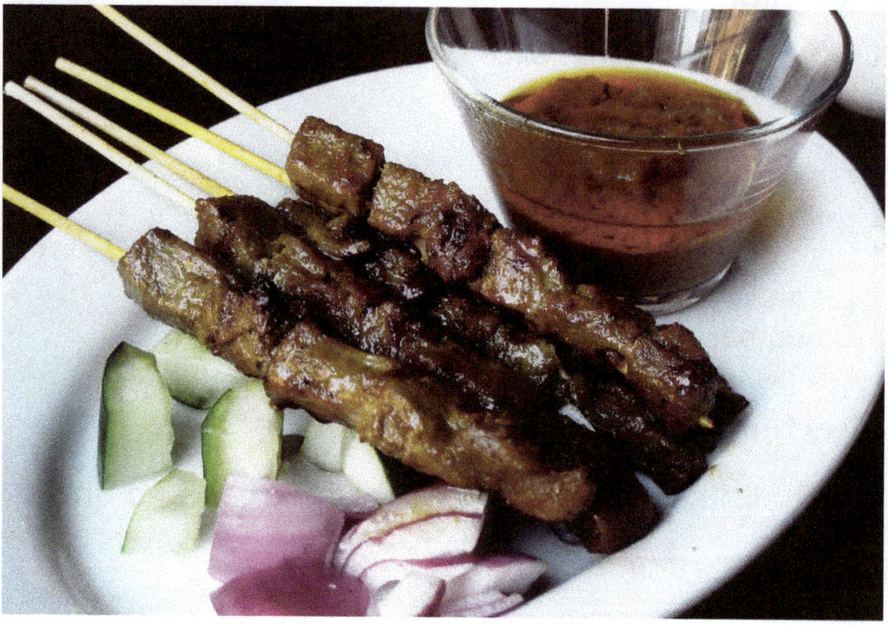

Steak Fajitas

Preparation Time:

10 minutes

Cooking Time:

15 minutes

Serve: 6

Ingredients:

1 lb steak, sliced
1/2 cup onion, sliced
1 red bell peppers, sliced
1 yellow bell peppers, sliced
1 green bell peppers, sliced
1 tbsp olive oil
1/4 tsp chili powder
1 tbsp fajita seasoning

Directions:

1.Add all ingredients large bowl and toss until well coated. Select Air Fry mode. Set time to 15 minutes and temperature 390 F then press START.

2.The air fryer display will prompt you to ADD FOOD once the temperature is reached then place fajita mixture in the air fryer basket. Stir after 10 minutes. Serve and enjoy.

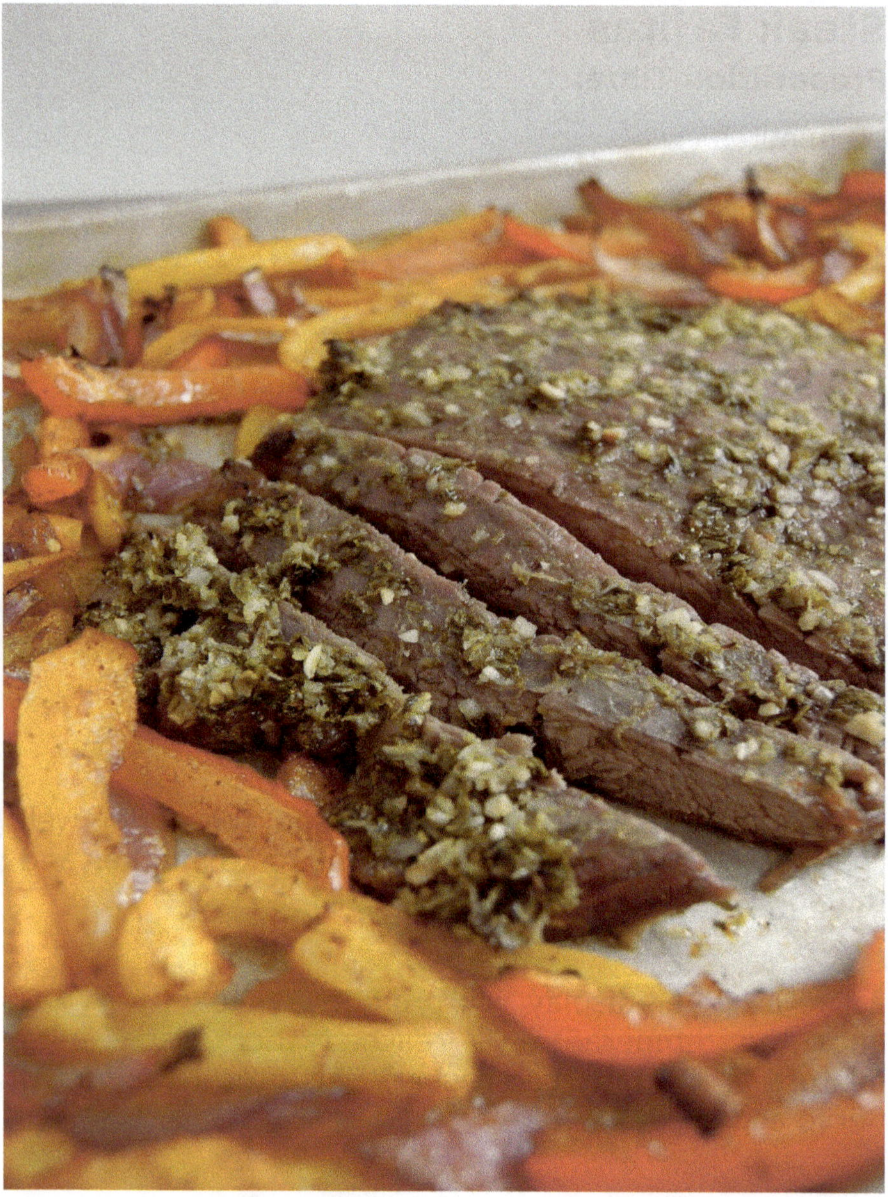

Buttery Steak Bites

Preparation Time:

10 minutes

Cooking Time:

7 minutes

Serve: 4

Ingredients:

1lb steak, cut into
1-inch cubes
2 tbsp steak seasoning
4 tbsp butter, melted
Pepper Salt

Directions:

1.Add steak, butter, seasoning, pepper, and salt into the bowl and mix well.

2.Select Air Fry mode. Set time to 7 minutes and temperature 350 F then press START.

3.The air fryer display will prompt you to ADD FOOD once the temperature is reached then add steak bites in the air fryer basket. Stir after 5 minutes. Serve and enjoy.

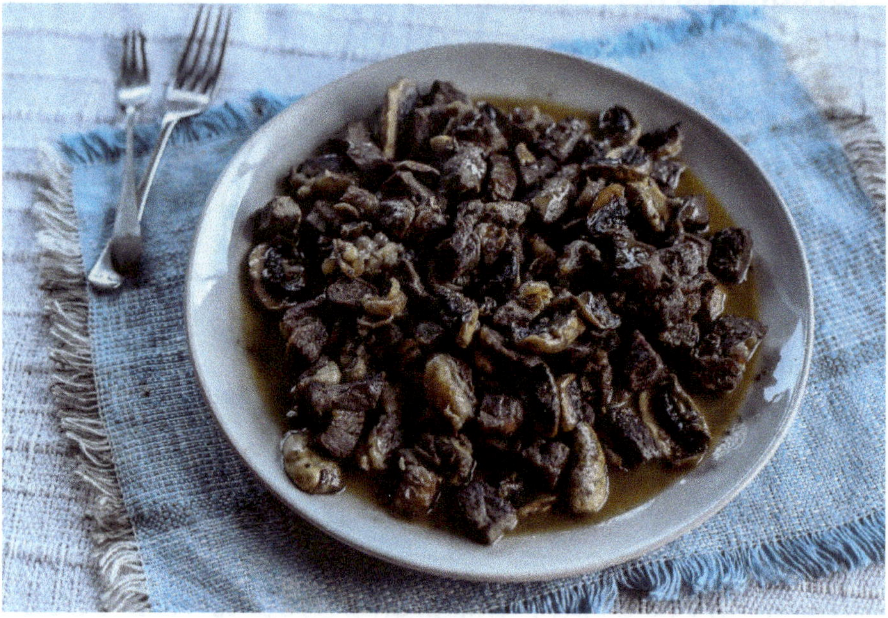

Greek Meatballs

Preparation Time:

10 minutes

Cooking Time:

20 minutes

Serve: 6

Ingredients:

1lbs ground pork
1 egg, lightly beaten
1 tbsp lemon zest
1/4 cup shallot, diced
1 tsp garlic powder
1 tsp dried oregano
1 tsp dried thyme
1/4 cup bell pepper, diced
1/4 cup yogurt
1 cup feta cheese, crumbled
1 cup spinach, cooked, squeezed & chopped
Pepper Salt

Directions:

1.Add all ingredients into the mixing bowl and mix until well combined.

2.Make small balls from the meat mixture.

3.Select Bake mode. Set time to 30 minutes and temperature 375 F then press START.

4.The air fryer display will prompt you to ADD FOOD once the temperature is reached then place meatballs in the air fryer basket. Stir halfway through. Serve and enjoy.

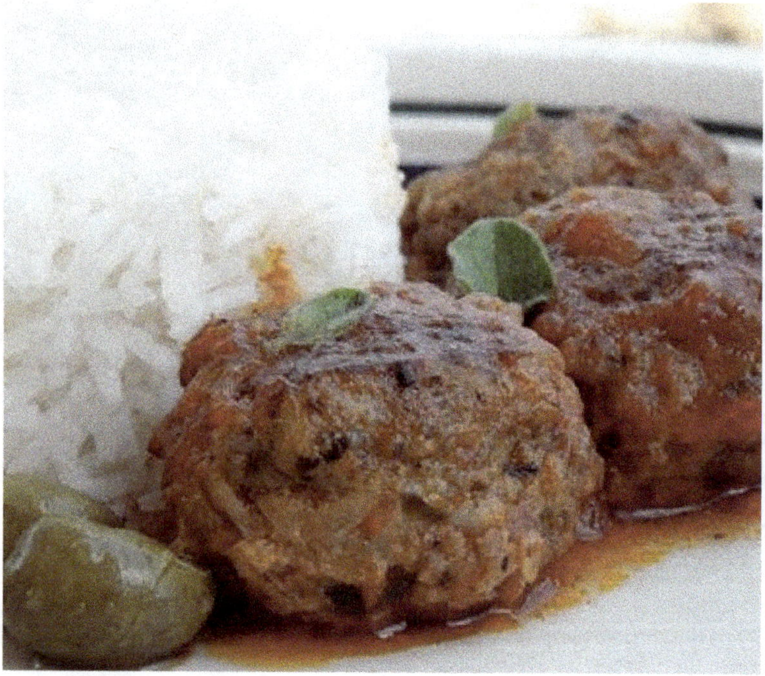

Pecan Crusted Pork Chops

Preparation Time:

10 minutes

Cooking Time:

20 minutes

Serve: 6

Ingredients:

1 1/2 lbs pork chops, boneless
2 eggs, lightly beaten
2 cups pecans, crushed
1/4 cup Dijon mustard

Directions:

1.Rub pork chops with mustard and set aside for 5 minutes.

2.In a shallow bowl, whisk eggs. In a separate shallow dish, add finely crushed pecans. Dip pork chops in egg and coat with crushed pecans.

3.Select Bake mode. Set time to 20 minutes and temperature 350 F then press START.

4.The air fryer display will prompt you to ADD FOOD once the temperature is reached then place pork chops in the air fryer basket. Serve and enjoy.

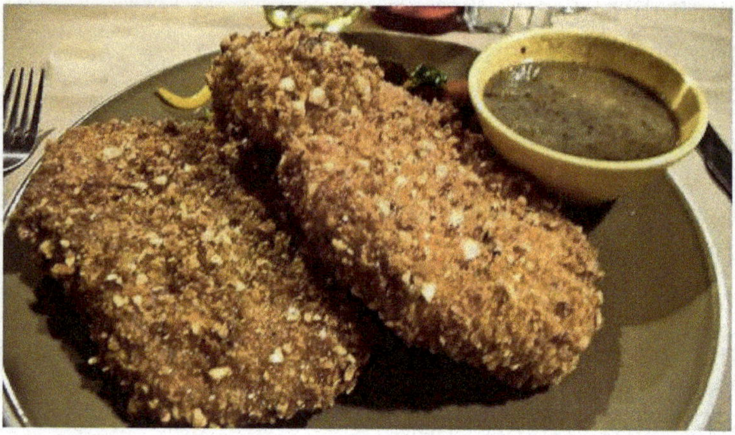

Asian Pork Steak

Preparation Time:

10 minutes

Cooking Time:

15 minutes

Serve: 4

Ingredients:

1lb pork steaks, boneless
1 tsp garam masala
1 tbsp ginger garlic paste
1/2 tsp cayenne
1/2 tsp ground cardamom
1 tsp cinnamon
1/2 onion, diced
1 tsp salt

Directions:

1.Add all ingredients except meat into the mixing bowl and mix well. Add the meat into the bowl and coat well.

2.Place meat into the refrigerator overnight. Select Air Fry mode. Set time to 15 minutes and temperature 330 F then press START.

3.The air fryer display will prompt you to ADD FOOD once the temperature is reached then place steaks in the air fryer basket. Turn halfway through. Serve and enjoy.

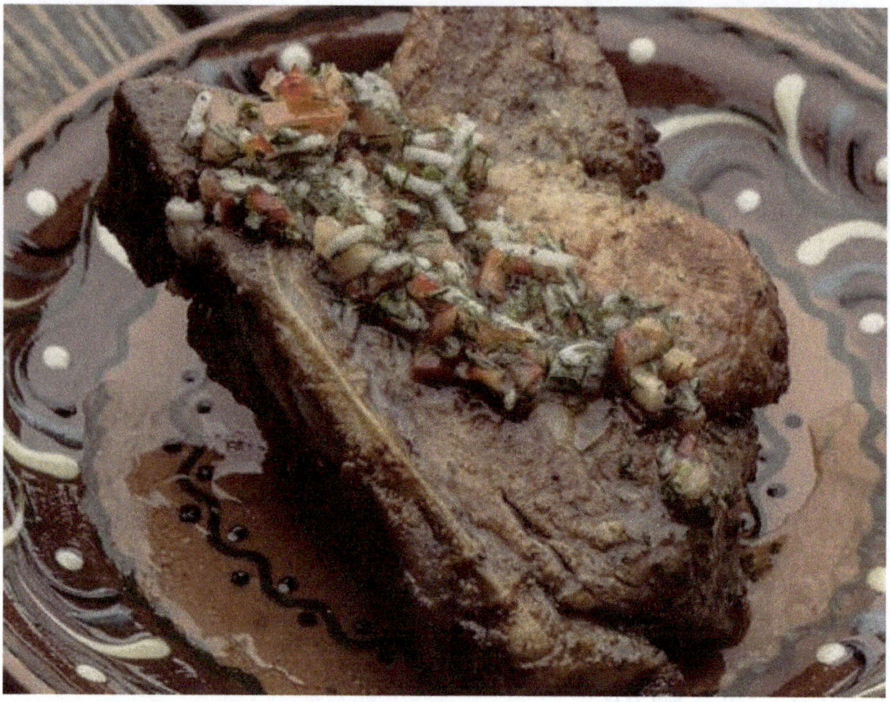

Serve Roasted Tomatoes with Cheese Topping

Cooking Time:

30 minutes

Servings:4

Ingredients:

½ cup cheddar cheese, shredded

¼ cup Parmesan cheese, grated

1 tsp olive oil

4 tomatoes, cut into

½ inch slices

2 tbsp parsley, chopped

Salt and black pepper to taste

Directions:

1.Preheat your Air Fryer to 380 F. Lightly salt the tomato slices and put them in the greased fryer basket in a single layer.

2.Top with mozzarella and Parmesan cheeses and sprinkle with black pepper. Air Fryer for 5-6 minutes until the cheese is melted and bubbly. Serve topped with parsley and enjoy!

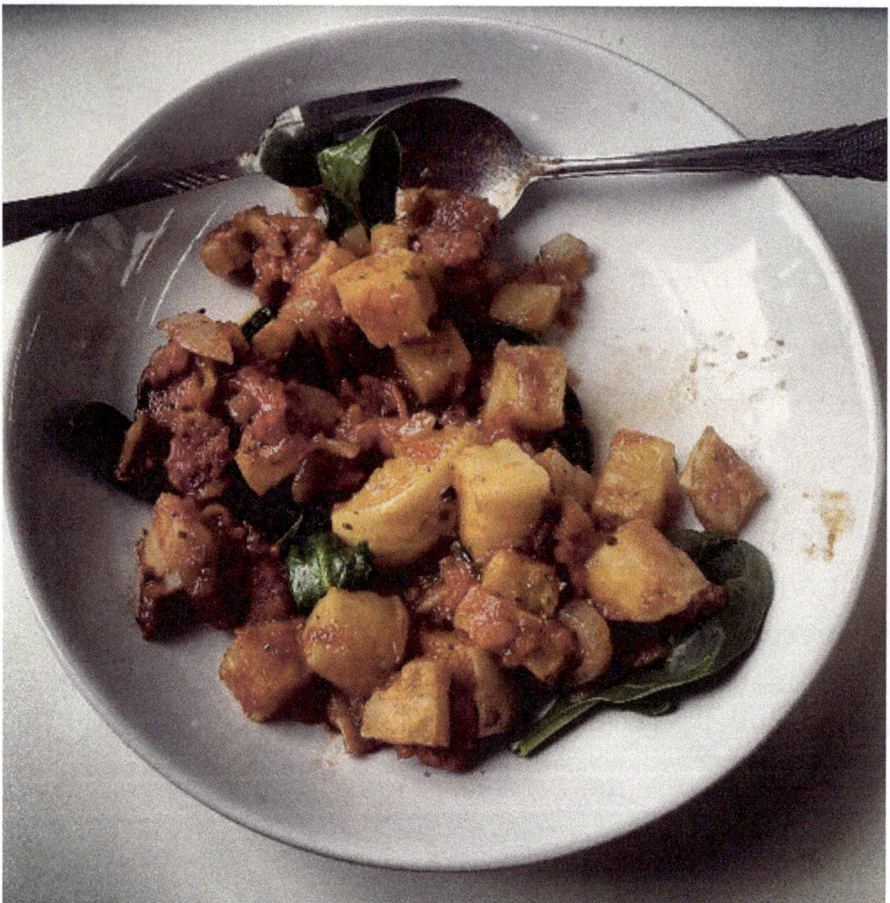

Curly Coconut Fries

Cooking Time:
20 minutes
Servings:2

Ingredients:

1potatoes, spiralized

1 tbsp tomato ketchup

2 tbsp olive oil

Salt and black pepper to taste

2 tbsp coconut oil

DIRECTIONS

1.air fryer to 360 F. In a bowl, coat potatoes with coconut oil, salt, and pepper.

2.Place in the frying basket and Air Fryer for 20 minutes, shaking once halfway through. Serve topped with mango sauce. enjoy!

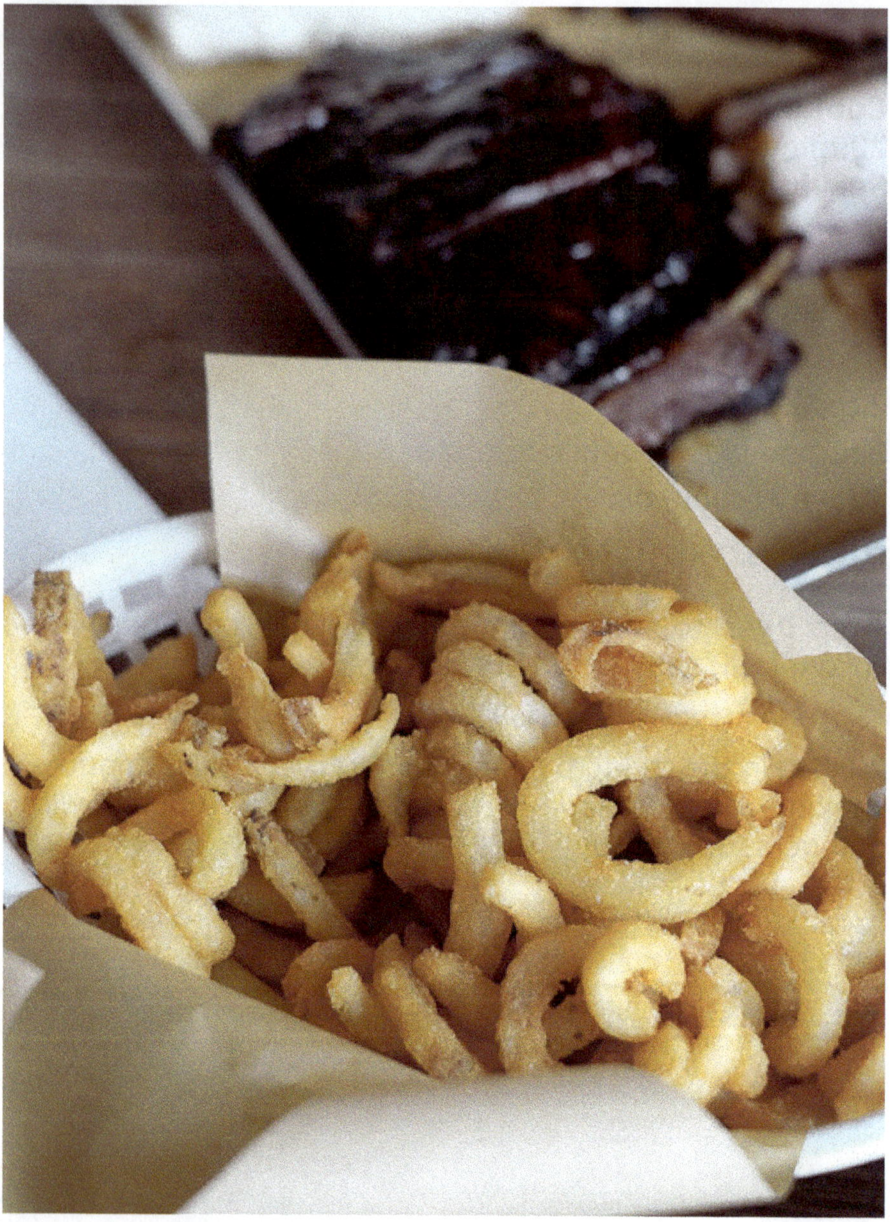

Crunchy Parmesan Zucchini

Cooking Time:
20 minutes
Servings:4

Ingredients:
4 small zucchinis, cut lengthwise
½ cup Parmesan cheese, grated
½ cup breadcrumbs
¼ cup melted butter
¼ cup fresh parsley, chopped
4 garlic cloves, minced
Salt and black pepper to taste

DIRECTIONS

1.Preheat air fryer to 370 F. In a bowl, mix breadcrumbs, Parmesan cheese, garlic, and parsley.

2.Season with salt and pepper and stir in the melted butter. Scoop out the seeds with a spoon. Spoon the mixture into the zucchini.

3.Arrange the zucchini on the greased frying basket and Bake for 12 minutes. Serve. enjoy!

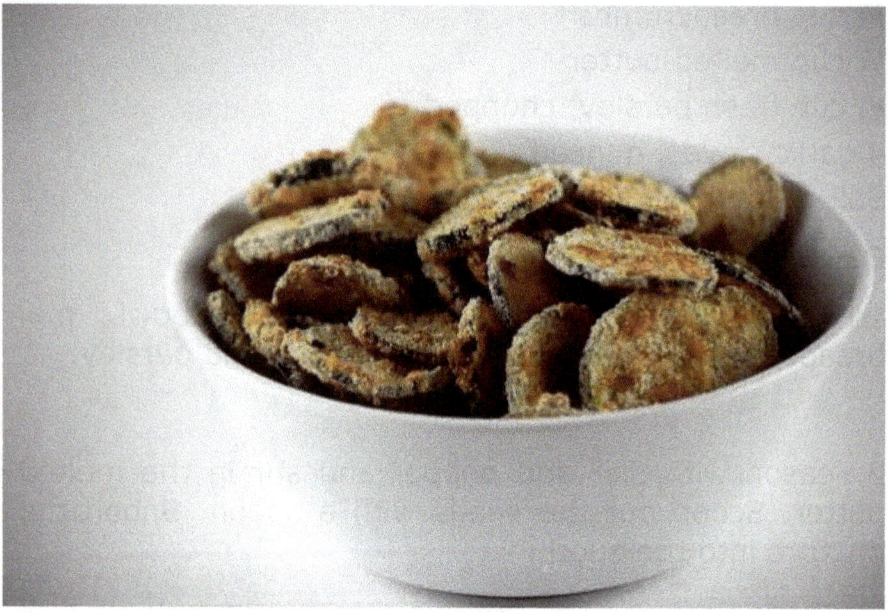

Avocado Fries with Pico de Gallo

Cooking Time:
30 minutes
Servings:4

Ingredients:

3 eggs, beaten in a bowl
4 avocados, cut in half, pits removed
2 tbsp olive oil
1 ½ cups panko breadcrumbs
1 ½ tsp paprika
Salt and black pepper to taste
2 tbsp cilantro, chopped
2 tomatoes, chopped
1 jalapeño pepper, minced
¼ cup red onions, finely chopped
1 lime, juiced 6 corn tortillas

Directions:

1.In a mixing bowl, thoroughly combine the cilantro, tomatoes, jalapeño pepper, red onion, lime juice, and salt.

2.Place in the fridge to allow the flavors to combine until ready to use. Preheat air fryer to 360 F. Remove the skin from the avocado, leaving the flesh intact.

3.Cut the halves into 5-6 lengthwise slices. Mix the breadcrumbs, salt, pepper, and paprika in a bowl.

4.Dip each avocado slice in the eggs, then in the panko mixture. Press the panko mixture gently into the avocado, so it sticks.

5.Put the avocado slices in a single layer on the greased fryer basket and brush with some olive oil. Air fry for 8-10 minutes, turning once until light brown and crispy. Serve with pico de gallo on the side. enjoy!

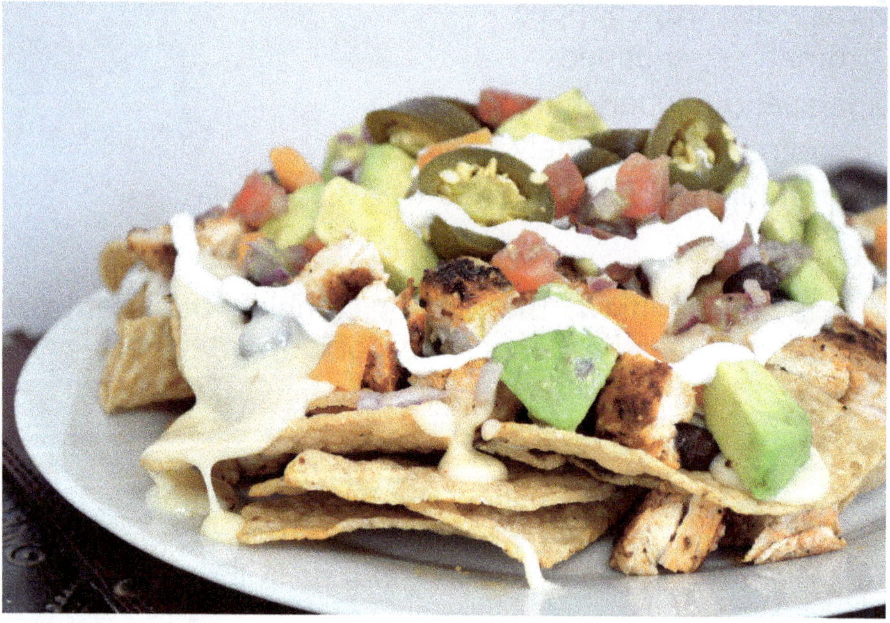

Broccoli with Parmesan Cheese

Cooking Time:
25 minutes
Servings:4

Ingredients:

1head broccoli, cut into florets

1 tbsp olive oil

Salt and black pepper to taste

1 oz Parmesan cheese, grated

Directions:

1.Preheat your air fryer to 360 F. In a bowl, mix all the ingredients.

2.Add the mixture to a greased baking dish and Bake in the air fryer for 20 minutes. Serve warm. enjoy!

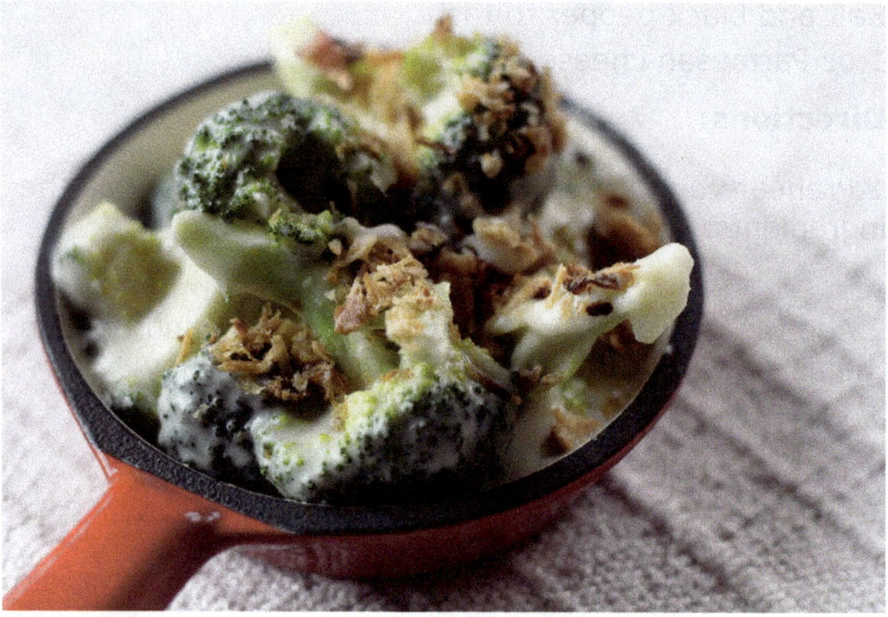

Roasted Balsamic Veggies

Cooking Time:
30 minutes
Servings:4

Ingredients:

1lb chopped veggies: potatoes, parsnips, zucchini, pumpkin, carrot, leeks

3tbsp olive oil

1tbsp balsamic vinegar

1 ntbsp agave syrup

Salt and black pepper to taste

DIRECTIONS

1.In a bowl, add olive oil, balsamic vinegar, agave syrup, salt, and black pepper; mix well.

2.Arrange the veggies on a baking tray and place them in the frying basket.

3.Drizzle with the dressing and massage with hands until well-coated. Air Fryer for 18-22 minutes at 360 F, tossing once halfway through. Serve. enjoy!

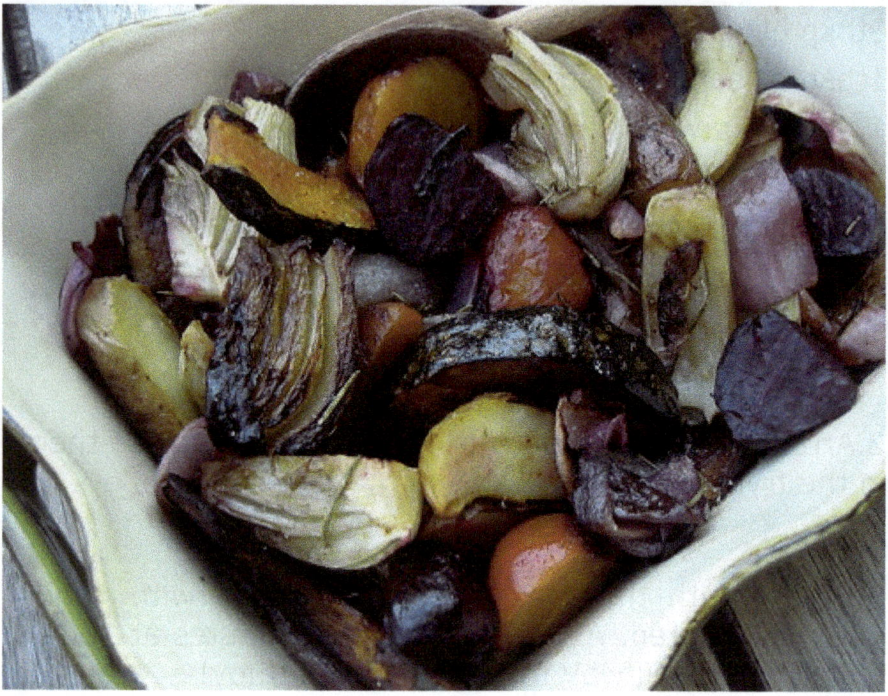

Middle Eastern Veggie Kofta

Cooking Time:

20 minutes

Servings:4

Ingredients:

2 tbsp corn flour
1 cup canned white beans
⅓ cup carrots, grated
2 potatoes, boiled and mashed
¼ cup fresh mint leaves, chopped
½ tsp ras el hanout powder
2 tbsp pine nuts
½ cup fresh mozzarella, chopped
3 garlic cloves, chopped
A bunch of skewers, soaked in water Salt to taste

DIRECTIONS

1.Preheat air fryer to 390 F. Place the beans, carrots, pine nuts, garlic, mozzarella, and mint in a food processor.

2.Blend until smooth, then transfer to a bowl. Add in the mashed potatoes, corn flour, salt, and ras el hanout and mix until fully incorporated.

3.Divide the mixture into equal shaped-patties, about 3 inches long by 1 inch thick.

4.Thread shapes on skewers and Bake in the greased frying basket for 10 minutes, turning once halfway through. Serve warm. enjoy!

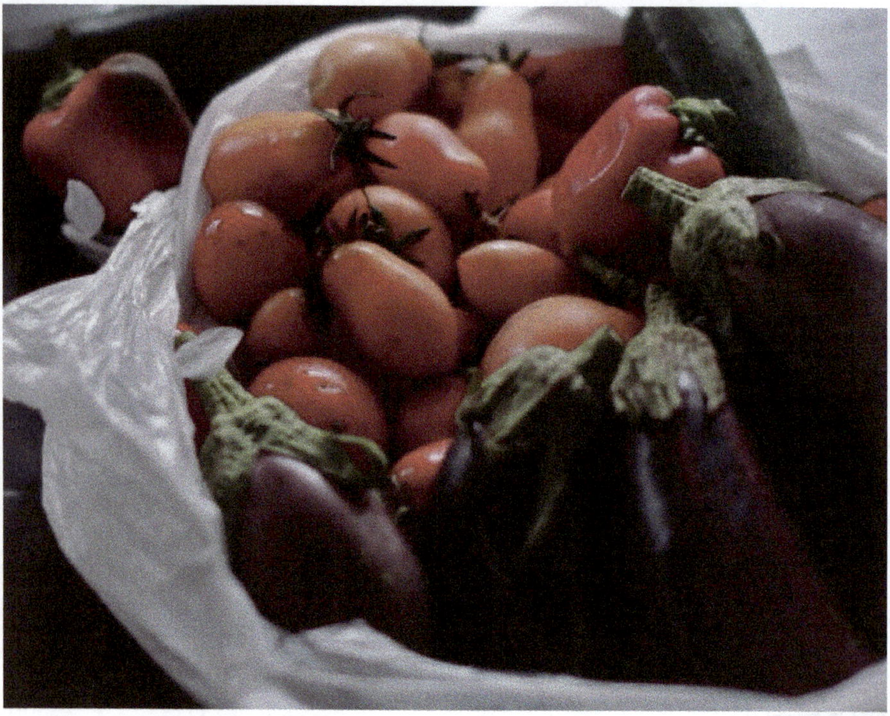

African Vegetables with Fontina Cheese

Cooking Time:

20 minutes

Servings:4

Ingredients:

2 tbsp olive oil
1 tsp cayenne pepper
2 tsp ground cumin
1 tbsp tomato purée
1 lemon, juiced
2 yellow bell peppers, cut into chunks
1 zucchini, sliced
1 eggplant, cut into chunks
1 red onion, cut into wedges
2 garlic cloves, minced
6 oz fontina cheese, grated
10 green olives

DIRECTIONS

1.Preheat air fryer to 370 F. In a small bowl, combine the cayenne pepper, garlic, ground cumin, tomato purée, lemon juice, and olive oil.

2.Add in the bell peppers, zucchini, eggplant, and onion and mix well.

3.Transfer to a baking dish and place in the air fryer. Bake for 18-20 minutes until golden. Sprinkle with fontina cheese and green olives and Bake for a further

5 minutes until the cheese is melted. Serve. enjoy!

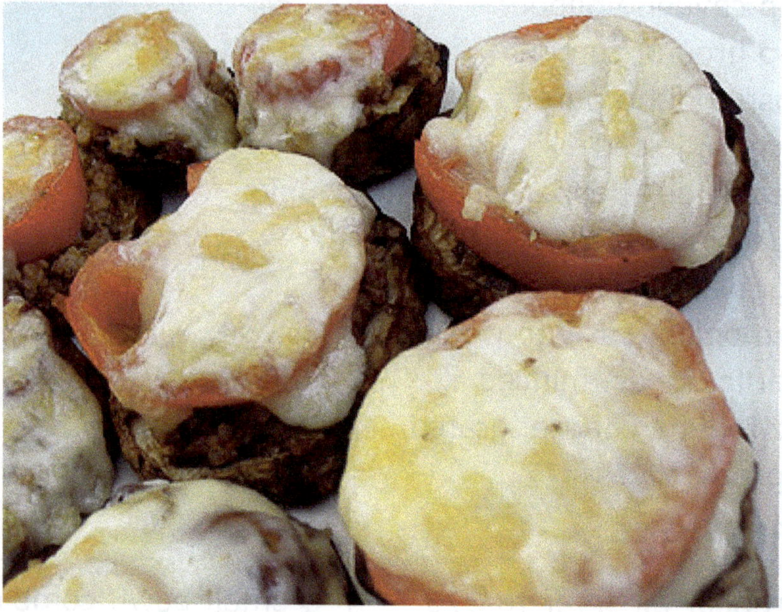

Egg & Cauliflower Rice Casserole

Cooking Time:

20 minutes

Servings:4

Ingredients:

1head cauliflower, cut into florets
2 tbsp olive oil
1 yellow bell pepper, chopped
1 cup okra, chopped
½ onion, chopped
Salt and black pepper to taste
1 tbsp soy sauce
2 eggs, beaten

Directions:

1.Preheat air fryer to 380 F. Grease a baking dish with cooking spray. Pulse cauliflower in a food processor until it resembles rice.

2.Add the cauli rice to the baking dish and mix in bell pepper, okra, onion, soy sauce, salt, and pepper.

3.Pour over the beaten eggs and drizzle with olive oil. Place the dish in the air fryer and Bake for 12 minutes. Serve warm. enjoy!

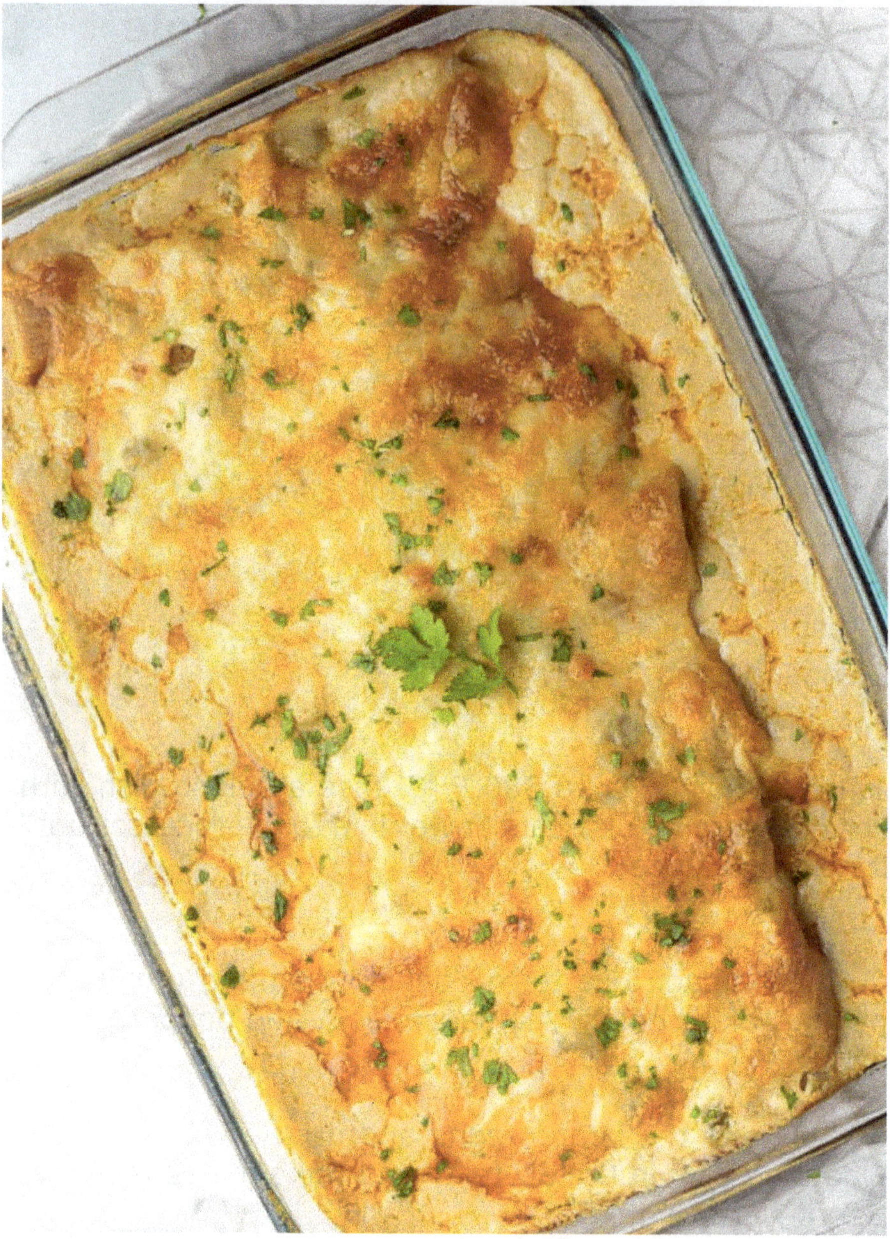

Cheesy English Muffins

Cooking Time:
15 minutes
Servings:2
Ingredients:

1English muffins, halved and toasted

½ cup cheddar cheese, shredded

1 ripe avocado, mashed

2 tbsp ranch-style salad dressing

½ cup alfalfa sprouts

1 tomato, chopped

½ sweet onion, chopped

1 tbsp sesame seeds, toasted

DIRECTIONS

1.Arrange the muffins open-faced in a greased baking dish.

2.Spread the mashed avocado on each half of the cupcakes. Top with sprouts, tomatoes, onion, dressing, and cheese.

3.Bake in the air fryer for 7-8 minutes at 350 F. Serve sprinkled with sesame seeds. enjoy!

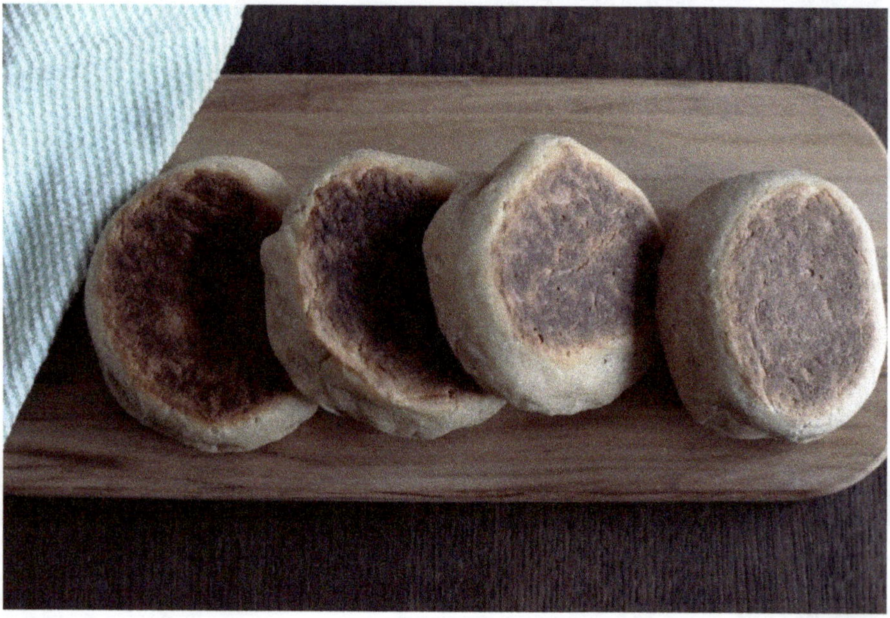

Romanian Polenta Fries

Cooking Time:
30 minutes
Servings:4

Ingredients:

2cups milk

1 cup instant polenta

Salt and black pepper to taste

2 tbsp fresh thyme, chopped

DIRECTIONS

1.Line a baking dish with parchment paper. Pour 2 cups of milk and 2 cups of water into a saucepan and let simmer.

2.Keep whisking as you pour in the polenta. Continue to whisk until polenta thickens and bubbles; season to taste.

3.Add polenta into the lined dish and spread out. Refrigerate for 45 minutes.

4.Slice the cold polenta into batons. Arrange the chips on the greased frying basket and AirFry for 14-16 minutes at 380 F, turning once halfway through. Make sure the fries are golden and crispy. Serve. enjoy!

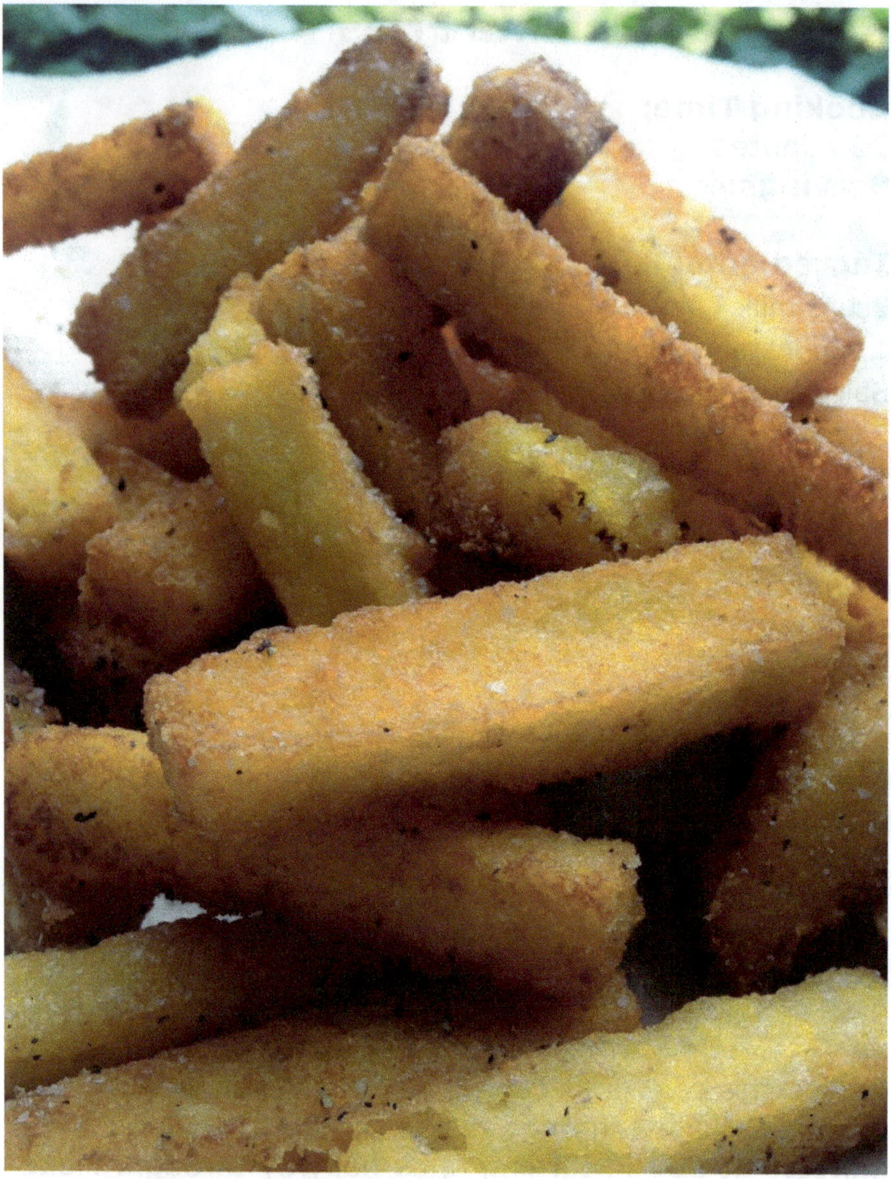

Mushroom Balls with Tomato Sauce

Cooking Time:
30 minutes
Servings:4

Ingredients:
⅓ cup cooked rice
1 lb mushrooms, chopped
½ onion, chopped
½ green bell peppers, chopped
Celery salt to taste
1 tbsp Worcestershire sauce
1 garlic clove, minced
2 cups tomato juice
1 tsp oregano

DIRECTIONS

1.In a food processor, blend the mushrooms until they resemble large crumbs. In a bowl, combine rice, ground mushrooms, onion, celery salt, green peppers, and garlic.

2.Shape into balls, and arrange them on the greased frying basket. Bake for 18 minutes at 370 degrees, shaking once.

3.In a saucepan over medium heat, pour tomato juice, oregano, celery salt, and Worcestershire sauce and cook until reduced by half. Pour the sauce over the balls and serve. enjoy!

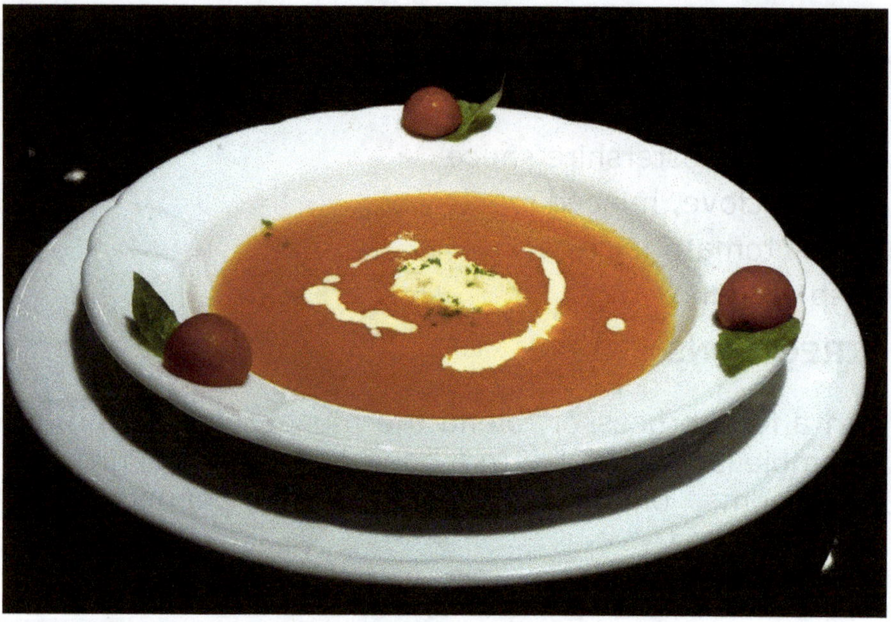

Brussels Sprouts with Garlic Aioli

Cooking Time:
25 minutes
Servings:4
Ingredients:

2garlic cloves, peel-on

1 lb Brussels sprouts, trimmed and halved

2 cups water

Salt and black pepper to taste

2 tbsp olive oil

2 tsp lemon juice

¾ cup mayonnaise

Directions:

1.Place a skillet over medium heat and roast the garlic cloves until lightly brown and fragrant.

2.Remove the skillet and place a pot with water; bring to a boil.

3.Blanch in Brussels sprouts for 3 minutes; drain. Preheat air fryer to 350 F. Drizzle the Brussels sprouts with olive oil and season with pepper and salt.

4.Pour them into frying basket and AirFry for 5 minutes, shaking once. Peel garlic and crush it in a bowl. Add in mayonnaise, lemon juice, black pepper, and salt; mix well.

5.Remove the Brussels sprouts onto a serving bowl and

serve with the garlic aioli. enjoy!

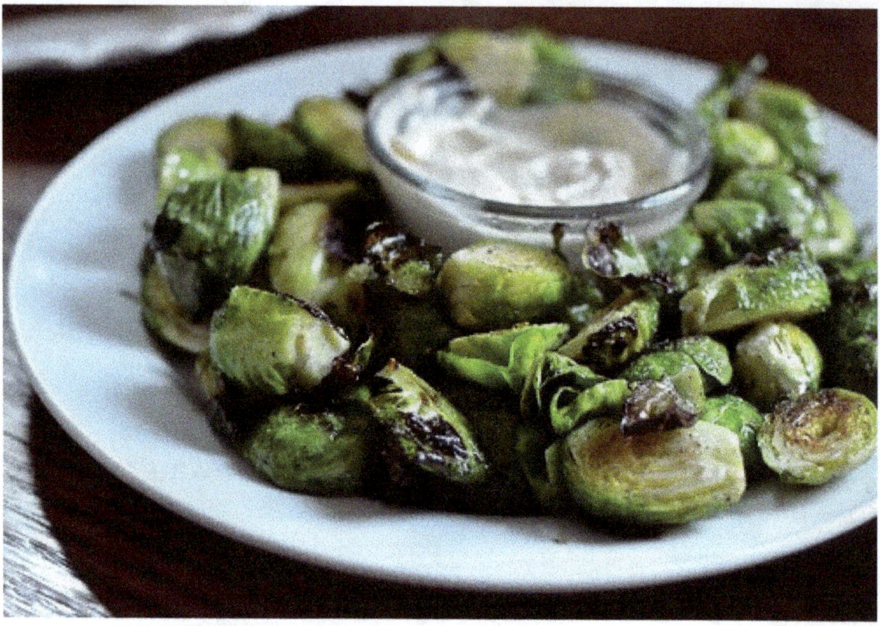

Eggplant Steaks with Garlic & Parsley

Cooking Time:
20 minutes
Servings:4

Ingredients:

2 eggplants, sliced
2 cups breadcrumbs
1 tsp Italian seasoning
1 cup flour
Salt to taste
4 eggs
2 garlic cloves, sliced
2 tbsp fresh parsley, chopped

DIRECTIONS

1.Preheat air fryer to 390 F. In a bowl, beat the eggs with salt. In a separate bowl, mix breadcrumbs and Italian seasoning.

2.In a third bowl, pour the flour. Dip eggplant steaks in the flour, followed by a dip in the eggs, and finally, coat in the breadcrumbs.

3.Place in the greased air fryer basket and Air Fryer for 10-12 minutes, flipping once. Remove to a platter and sprinkle with garlic and parsley to serve. enjoy!

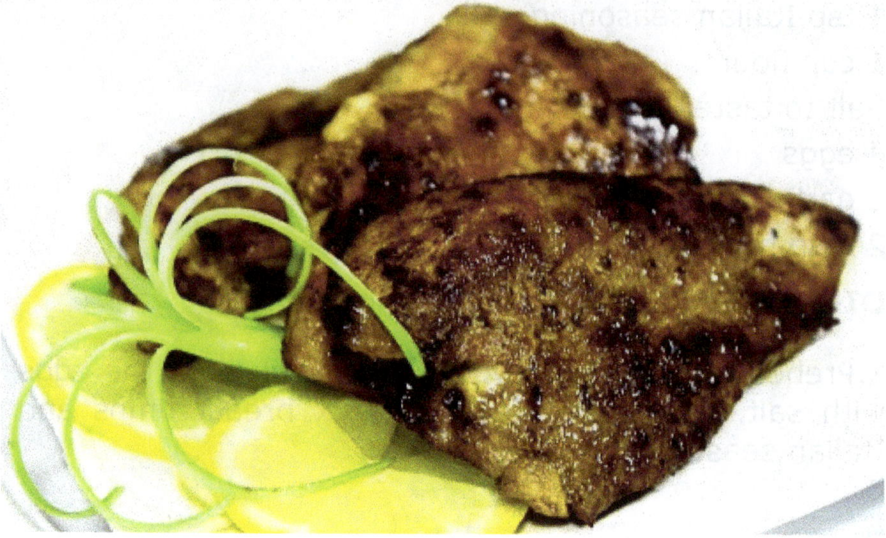

Breaded Italian Green Beans

Cooking Time:
20 minutes
Servings:4

Ingredients:

1cup panko breadcrumbs

2 eggs, beaten

½ cup Parmesan cheese, grated

½ cup flour

1 tsp cayenne pepper

1 ½ lb green beans

1 cup tomato pasta sauce

Salt and black pepper to taste

Directions:

1.Preheat air fryer to 400 F. In a bowl, mix breadcrumbs, Parmesan cheese, cayenne pepper, salt, and pepper.

2.Coat the green beans in the flour, followed by the beaten egg and finally the Parmesan-panko crumbs. Air Fryer in the fryer for 15 minutes, turning once halfway through. Serve with tomato sauce. enjoy!

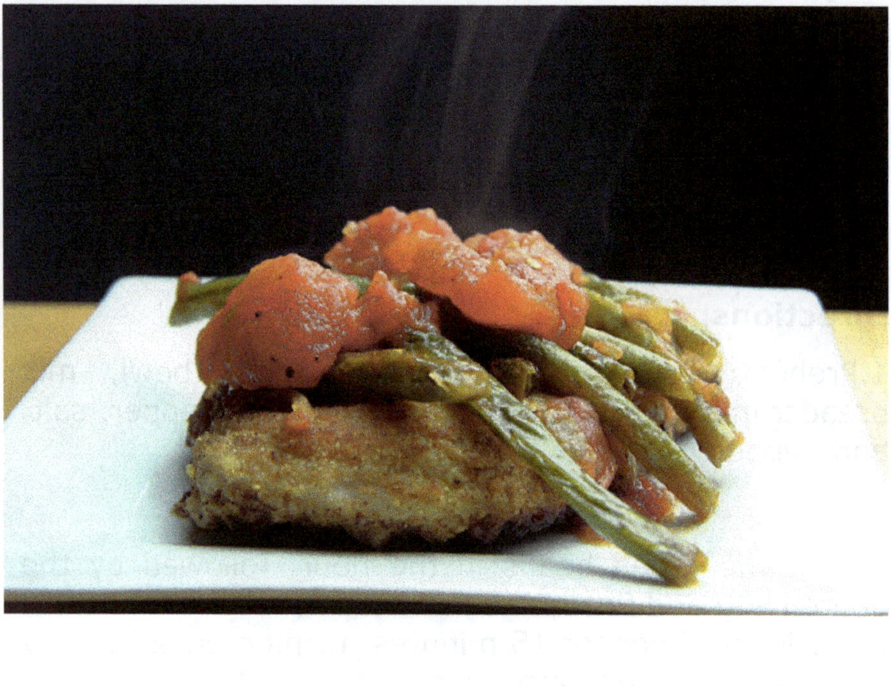

Tempura Veggies with Sesame Soy Sauce

Cooking Time:
20 minutes
Servings:4

Ingredients:

1lb chopped veggies carrot, parsnip, green beans, zucchini, onion rings, asparagus, cauliflower

1 ½ cups plain flour

Salt and black pepper to taste

1 ½ tbsp cornstarch

¾ cup cold water

Dipping sauce:

4 tbsp soy sauce Juice of 1 lemon

½ tsp sesame oil

½ tsp sugar

½ garlic clove, chopped

½ tsp sweet chili sauce

DIRECTIONS

1.Line the air fryer basket with baking paper. In a bowl, mix flour, salt, pepper, and cornstarch; whisk to combine.

2.Keep whisking as you add in water, so a smooth batter is formed. Dip each veggie piece into the batter and place it into the frying basket.

3.AirFry for 12 minutes at 360 F, turning once; cook until crispy. Mix all dipping ingredients in a bowl. Serve with the crispy veggies. enjoy!

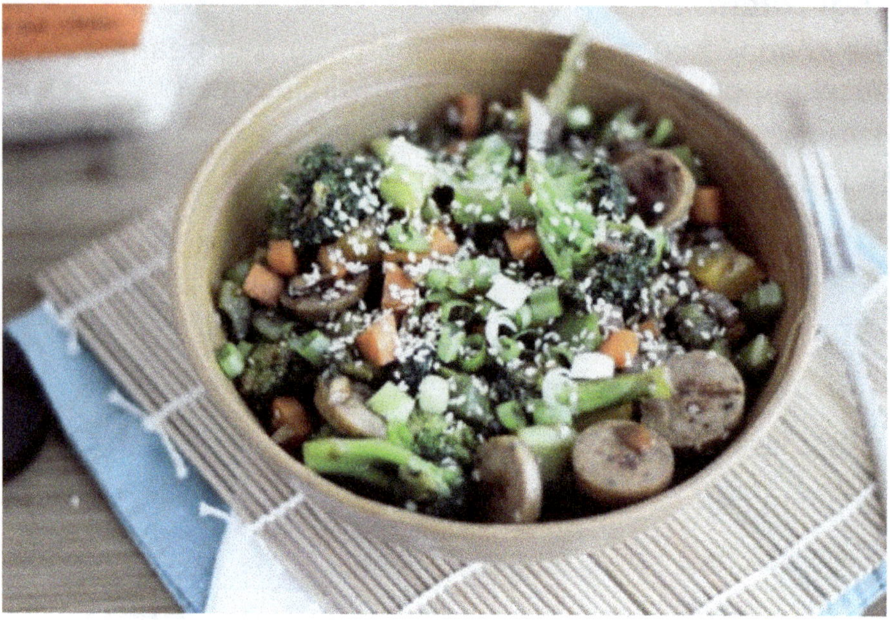

Turmeric Crispy Chickpeas

Cooking Time:
20 minutes
Servings:4

Ingredients:

1 15-oz can chickpeas, rinsed

1 tbsp butter, melted

½ tsp dried rosemary

¼ tsp turmeric

DIRECTIONS

1.Preheat air fryer to 380 F. In a bowl, combine together chickpeas, butter, rosemary, turmeric, and salt; toss to coat.

2.Place the in the greased frying basket and Air Fryer for 6 minutes. Shake, and cook for 6 more minutes until crispy. enjoy!

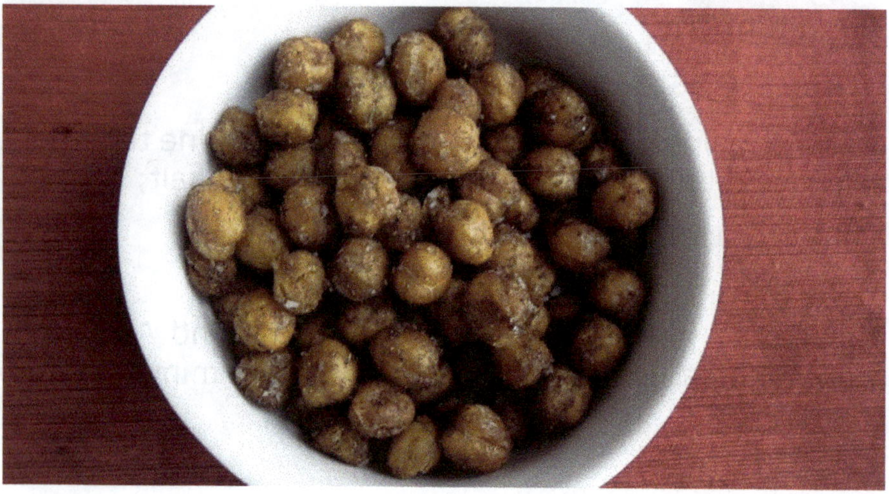

Easy Vegetable Croquettes

Cooking Time:
45 minutes
Servings:4

Ingredients:

1 lb red potatoes
1 ¼ cups milk
Salt to taste
3 tbsp butter
2 tsp olive oil
1 red bell pepper, chopped
½ cup baby spinach, chopped
½ lb mushrooms, chopped
½ lb broccoli florets, chopped
1 green onion, sliced
1 red onion, chopped
2 garlic cloves, minced
1 carrot, grated
⅓ cup flour
2 eggs, beaten
1 ½ cups breadcrumbs

DIRECTIONS

1.Cover the potatoes with salted water in a pot over medium heat and cook for about 15-18 minutes. Drain and place in a bowl.

2.Add in 2 tbsp of butter, 1 cup of milk, and salt. Mash with a potato masher.

3.In a food processor, place onion, garlic, bell pepper, broccoli, mushrooms, green onion, spinach, olive oil, salt, and remaining milk and pulse until a breadcrumb texture is formed.

4.Mix with mashed potatoes. Using your hands, create oblong balls out of the mixture and place them on a baking sheet in a single layer. Refrigerate for 30 minutes.

5.Preheat air fryer to 390 F. Take 3 separate bowls, pour breadcrumbs in one, flour in another, and eggs in a third bowl. Remove the croquettes from the fridge.

6.Dredge the croquettes in flour, then in the eggs, and finally in the crumbs. Arrange them on the greased frying basket without overlapping.

7.AirFry for 12-14 minutes, shaking once. Remove to a wire rack. Let cool and serve. enjoy!

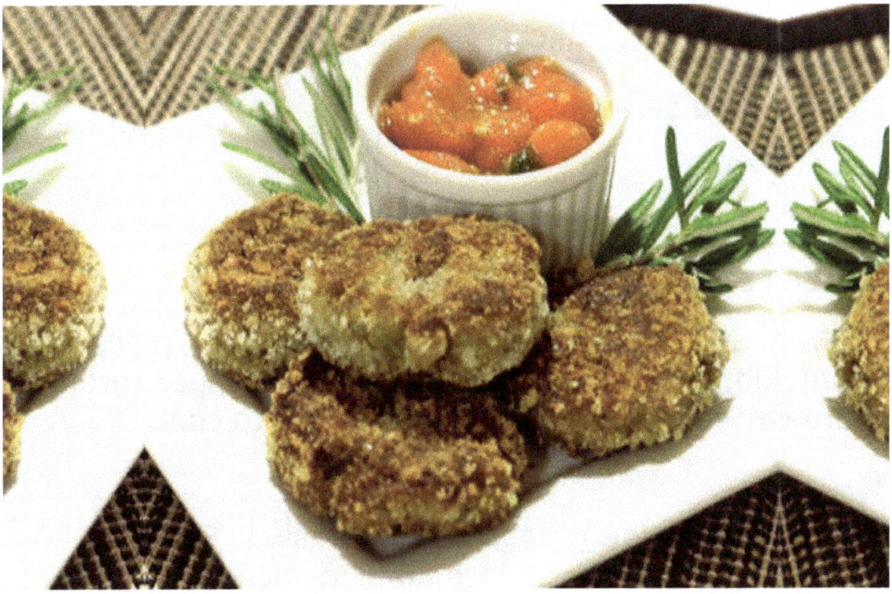

Chili Roasted Pumpkin with Orzo

Cooking Time:
35 minutes
Servings:4

INGREDIENTS

1lb pumpkin, peeled and cubed

red bell peppers, diced

2 shallots, quartered

1 red chili pepper, minced

1 tsp ground caraway seeds

1 cup orzo

Salt and black pepper to taste

DIRECTIONS

1.Preheat air fryer to 380 F. In a bowl, place the pumpkin, bell peppers, shallots, chili pepper, ground caraway seeds, salt, and pepper; toss to coat.

2.Transfer to the greased frying basket. Bake for 20-25 minutes, shaking once until golden. Place a pot filled with salted water over medium heat and bring to a boil.

3.Add in the orzo and cook for 4 minutes. Drain and place on a serving platter. Spread the baked pumpkin all over. Serve and enjoy!

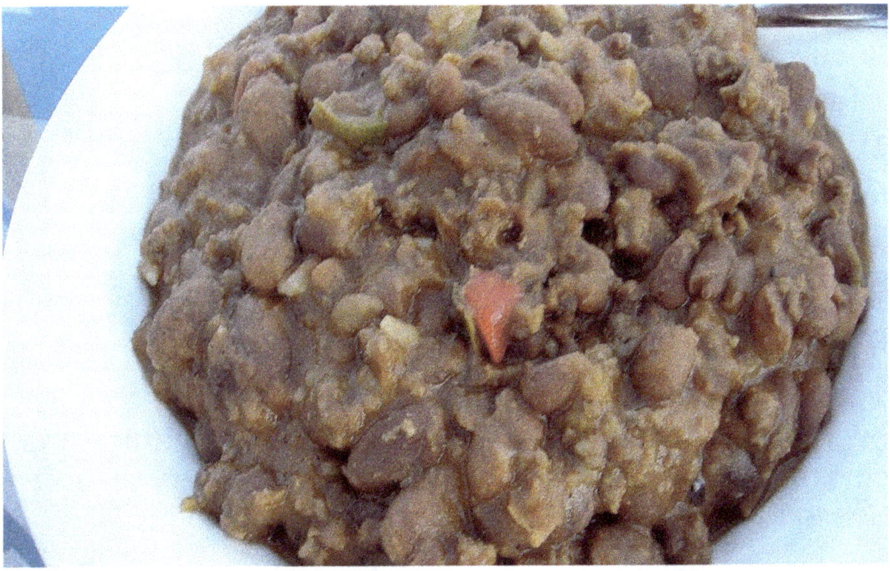

Vegetable & Goat Cheese Tian

Cooking Time:
35 minutes
Servings:4

Ingredients:

tbsp butter

1 garlic clove, minced

2 tomatoes, sliced

1 cup canned chickpeas, drained

¼ cup black olives, pitted and chopped

1 fennel bulb, sliced

1 zucchini, sliced into rounds

4 oz goat cheese, sliced into rounds

1 tsp dried thyme

Salt and black pepper to taste

Directions:

1.Preheat air fryer to 360 F. Melt the butter in a skillet over medium heat and sauté the fennel, garlic, and chickpeas for 5-6 minutes, stirring often until soft. Season with thyme, salt, and pepper.

2.Transfer to a baking dish and arrange tomato, zucchini, and cheese slices on top. Scatter with black olives.

3.Place the dish in the fryer and Bake for 20-25 minutes until the cheese is melted and golden. Remove and let sit for a few minutes before serving. enjoy!

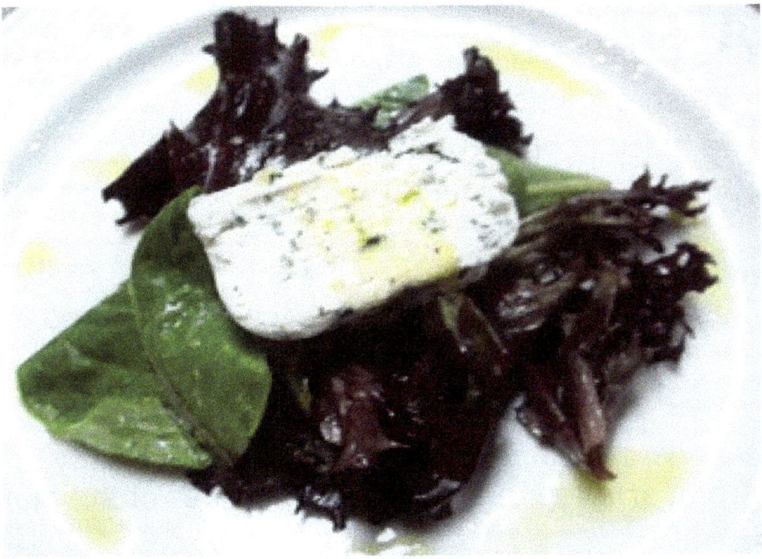

Questa foto di Autore sconosciuto è concesso in licenza da CC BY-SA

Dilled Zucchini Egg Cakes

Cooking Time:
25 minutes
Servings:4

Ingredients:

12 oz thawed puff pastry

4 large eggs

1 medium zucchini, sliced

4 oz feta cheese, drained and crumbled

2 tbsp fresh dill, chopped

Salt and black pepper to taste

DIRECTIONS

1.Preheat air fryer to 360 F. In a bowl, whisk the eggs with salt and pepper. Stir in zucchini, dill, and feta cheese.

2.Grease a muffin tin tray with cooking spray. Roll pastry and arrange them to cover the sides of the muffin holes.

3.Divide the egg mixture evenly between the holes. Place the muffin tray in your air fryer and Bake for 13-15 minutes, until golden. enjoy!

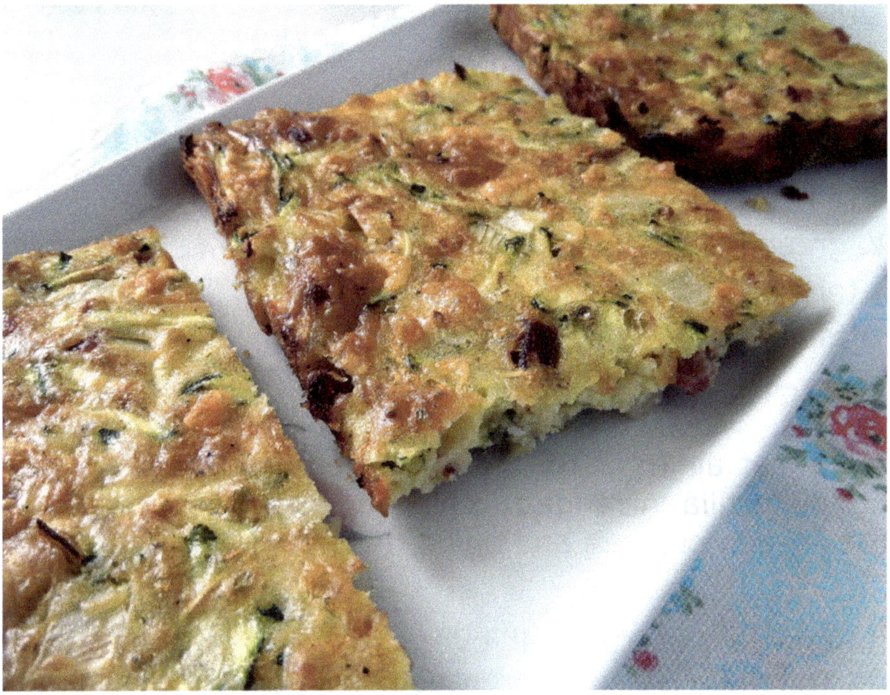

Vegetable Tortilla Pizza

Cooking Time:
15 minutes
Servings:4
Ingredients:

¼ tbsp tomato paste

1 tbsp cheddar cheese, grated

1 tbsp mozzarella cheese, grated

1 tbsp cooked sweet corn

4 zucchini slices

4 eggplant slices

4 red onion rings

½ green bell pepper, chopped

1 tortilla

¼ tsp basil

DIRECTIONS

1.Preheat air fryer to 350 F. Spread the tomato paste on the tortilla. Arrange zucchini and eggplant slices first, then green peppers and onion rings.

2.Sprinkle the corn all over. Top with cheddar and mozzarella. Place on a greased baking tray and fit in the fryer.

3.Bake for 10-12 minutes. Sprinkle with basil to serve. enjoy!

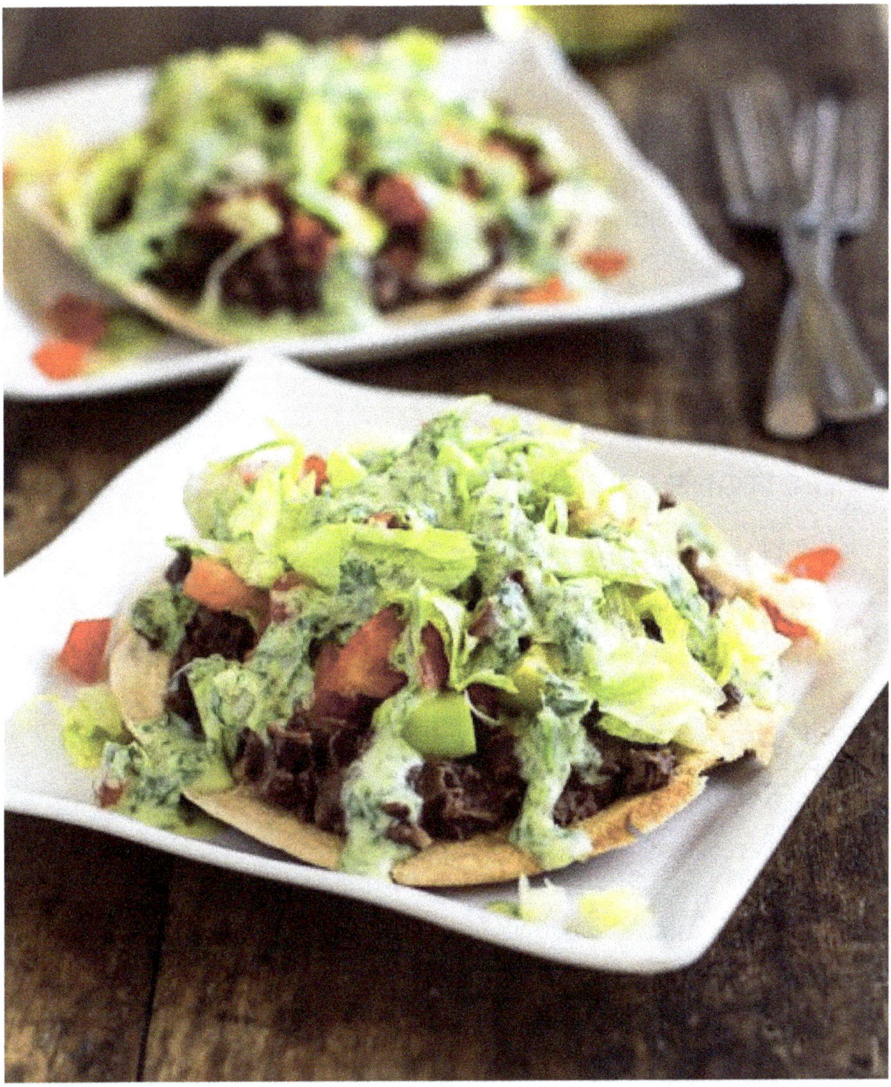

Easy Fried Green Tomatoes

Cooking Time:
15 minutes
Servings:2

Ingredients:
1 green tomato, sliced
¼ tbsp creole seasoning
Salt and black pepper to taste
¼ cup flour
½ cup buttermilk
1 cup breadcrumbs

DIRECTIONS

1.Add flour to one bowl and buttermilk to another. Season tomatoes with salt and pepper. Make a mix of creole seasoning and breadcrumbs.

2.Roll tomato slices up in the flour, dip in buttermilk, and then into the breadcrumbs.

3.AirFry in the greased frying basket for 5 minutes at 400 F, turning once. enjoy!

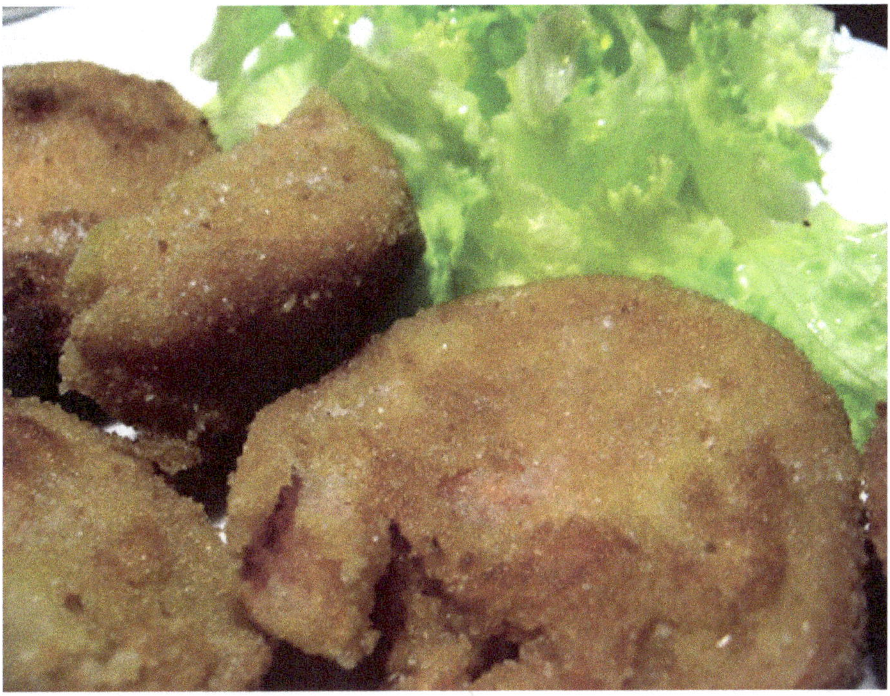

Honey Baby Carrots

Cooking Time:
20 minutes
Servings:4

Ingredients:
1 lb Baby carrots
1 tsp dried dill
2 tbsp olive oil
1 tbsp honey
Salt and black pepper to taste

DIRECTIONS

1.Preheat air fryer to 350 F. In a bowl, mix olive oil, carrots, and honey; stir to coat.

2.Season with dill, pepper, and salt. Place coated carrots in the greased frying basket and Air Fry for 12 minutes, shaking once. Serve warm or chilled. enjoy!

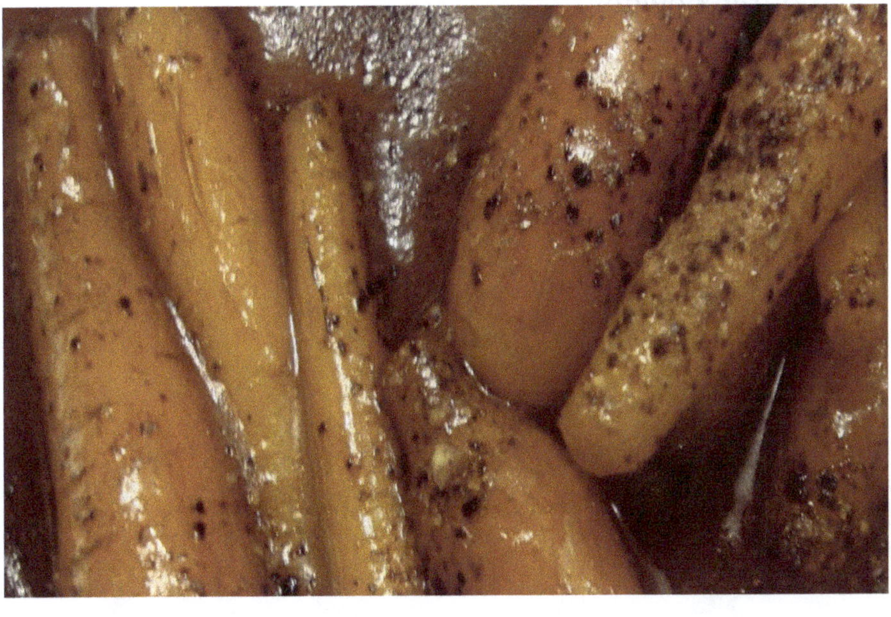

Homemade Cipollini Onions

Cooking Time:
20 minutes
Servings:4

Ingredients:

1lb cipollini onions, cut into flowers

2 tbsp olive oil

1 tsp cayenne pepper

1 tsp garlic powder

2 cups flour

Salt and black pepper to taste

1 tbsp paprika

¼ cup mayonnaise

1 tbsp ketchup

¼ cup mayonnaise

¼ cup sour cream

Directions:

1.Preheat your air fryer to 360 F. In a bowl, mix salt, pepper, paprika, flour, garlic powder, and cayenne pepper.

2.Stir in mayonnaise, ketchup, and sour cream. Coat the onions with the prepared mixture and spray with olive oil. Add the coated onions to a baking dish and Bake in the air fryer for 15 minutes. enjoy!

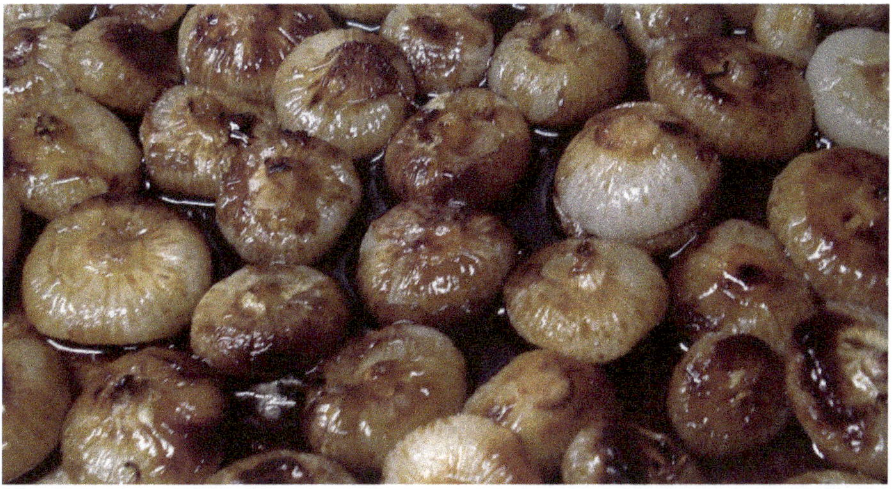

Party Crispy Nachos

Cooking Time:
30 minutes
Servings:2

Ingredients:

1 cup sweet corn

1 cup all-purpose flour

1 tbsp butter

½ tsp chili powder

Salt to taste

Directions:

1.Add a small amount of water to the sweet corn and grind until you obtain a very fine paste. In a bowl, mix flour, salt, chili powder, and butter; add corn and stir.

2.Knead with your palm until you obtain a stiff dough. Preheat air fryer to 350 F. On a working surface, dust a little bit of flour and spread the dough with a rolling pin.

3.Make it around ½ inch thick. Cut into tringle-shape and Air Fryer in the greased frying basket for around 10 minutes. Serve with guacamole salsa. enjoy!

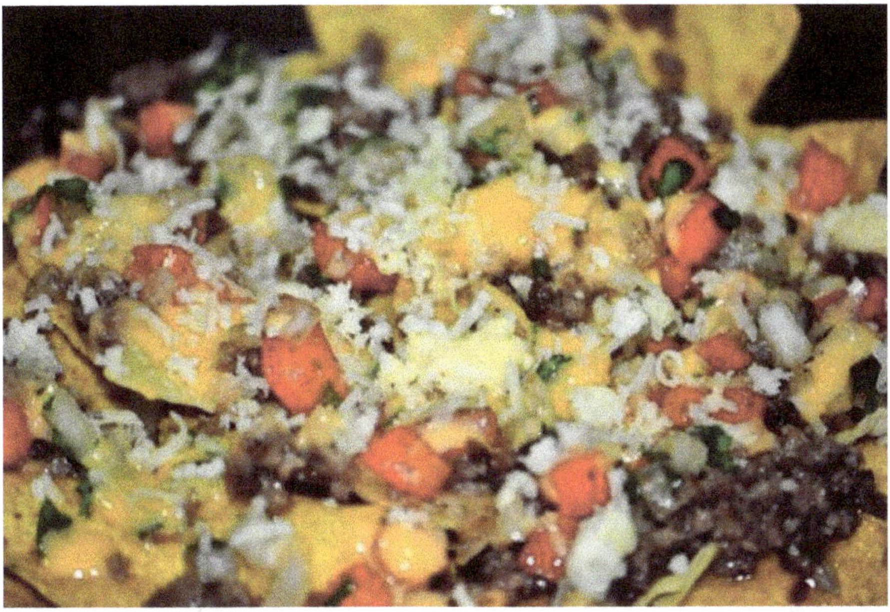

Green Vegetable Rotini Pasta Bake

Cooking time:
30 minutes
Servings:4
Ingredients:

1 cup green peas

1 lb broccoli florets, steamed

1 cup kale, chopped

1 garlic clove, minced

2 tbsp flour

2 cups milk

¼ cup mozzarella cheese, grated

16 oz rotini pasta

3 tbsp butter

1 tbsp fresh basil, chopped

Salt and black pepper to taste

DIRECTIONS

1.Bring a large saucepan of salted water to a boil. Add in the rotini pasta and cook following pack instructions.

2.Drain and set aside. Melt butter in a skillet over medium heat and sauté garlic for 1 minute. Stir in flour for 1 minute.

3.Gradually add in the milk and simmer until slightly thickened, 3 minutes.

4.Preheat air fryer to 350 F. Transfer the milk mixture to a baking dish and add in the pasta, broccoli, kale, green peas, salt, and pepper; stir to combine.

5.Top with the mozzarella cheese and sprinkle with basil. Place in the air fryer and Bake for 10-12 minutes until the cheese is golden. Serve warm. enjoy!

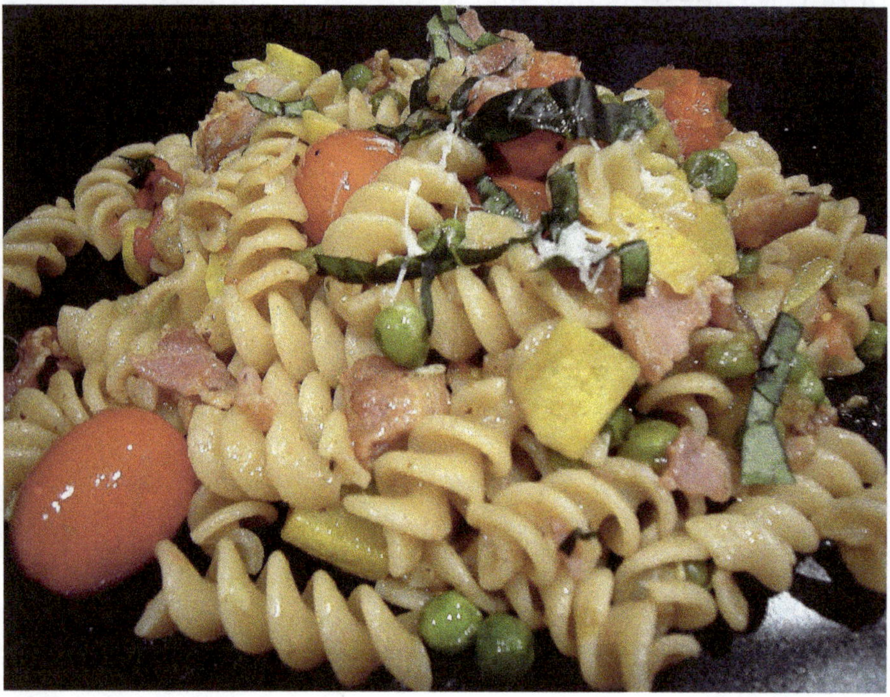

Tomato Sandwiches with Feta & Pesto

Cooking Time:
25 minutes
Servings:2

Ingredients:

1 heirloom tomato

1 4-oz block Feta cheese

1 small red onion, thinly sliced

1 garlic clove

Salt to taste

2 tsp + ¼ cup olive oil

1 ½ tbsp pine nuts, toasted

2 tbsp fresh parsley, chopped

¼ cup Parmesan cheese, grated

¼ cup fresh basil, chopped

DIRECTIONS

1.Add basil, pine nuts, garlic, Parmesan cheese, and salt to a food processor. Pulse while slowly adding ¼ cup of olive oil. Preheat air fryer to 390 F.

2.Slice feta cheese and tomato into ½-inch slices. Spread the obtained pesto sauce on the tomato slices. Top with feta cheese and onion and drizzle the remaining olive oil.

3.Place the tomato in the greased frying basket and Bake for 6-8 minutes. Remove to a serving platter, sprinkle lightly with salt, and top with fresh parsley.

Serve chilled. enjoy!

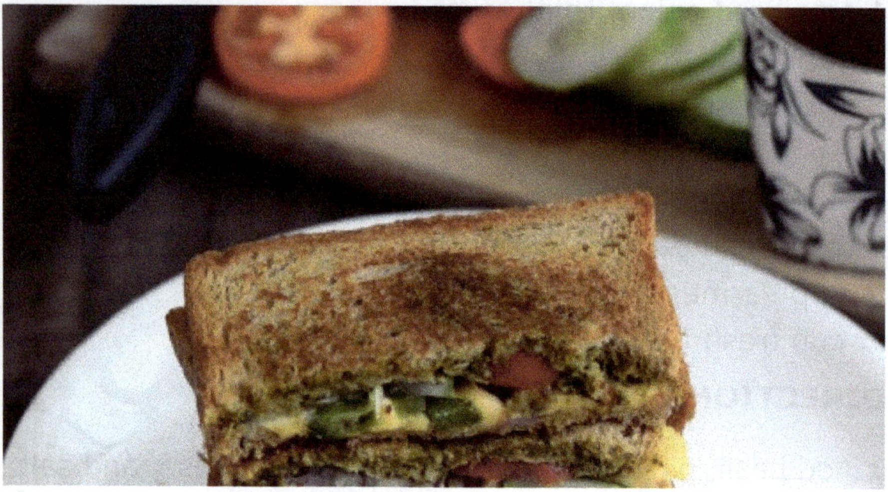

Homemade Pie with Root Vegetables

Cooking Time:

40 minutes

Servings:4

Ingredients:

1 lb potatoes, cubed
3 tbsp pine nuts
1 parsnip, chopped
½ cup Parmesan cheese, grated
1 cup crème fraiche
1 bread slice, diced
½ tsp dried sage
2 tbsp butter
1 tsp yellow mustard

DIRECTIONS

1.Boil potatoes and parsnip in a pot filled with salted water over medium heat for 15 minutes. Drain and place in a bowl.

2.Add in mustard, crème fraiche, sage, butter, salt, and pepper and mash them using a potato masher. Mix in bread and Parmesan cheese.

3.Preheat air fryer to 360 F. Add the resulting batter to a greased baking dish and place it in the air fryer. Bake for 15 minutes. Serve warm or chilled. enjoy!

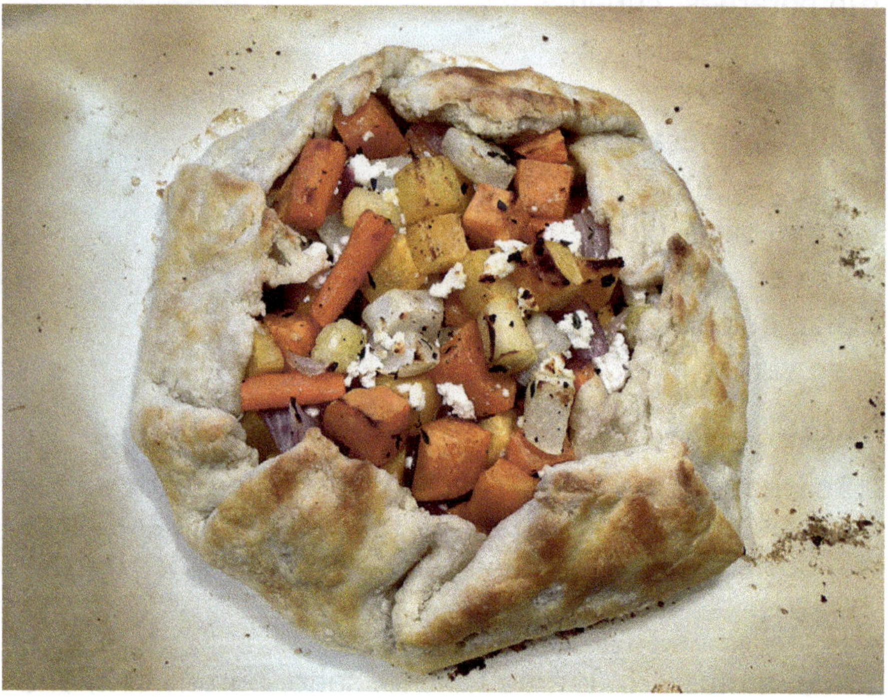

Baked Mediterranean Shakshuka

Cooking Time:
25 minutes
Servings:4

Ingredients:
1 onion, sliced
2 garlic cloves, minced
2 tbsp olive oil
1 tsp ground cumin
2 tsp paprika
¼ tsp chili powder
1 red bell pepper, seeded and diced
2 14.5-oz cans tomatoes, diced
4 eggs
2 tbsp fresh parsley, chopped
4 tbsp feta cheese, crumbled
Salt and black pepper to taste

Directions:

1.Heat olive oil in a skillet over medium heat and sauté bell pepper, onion, and garlic for 5 minutes until tender.

2.Stir in paprika, chili powder, cumin, salt, and pepper and pour in the tomatoes. Simmer for 10 minutes and transfer to a baking pan. Crack in the eggs. Bake in the air fryer for 12 minutes at 370 F enjoy!

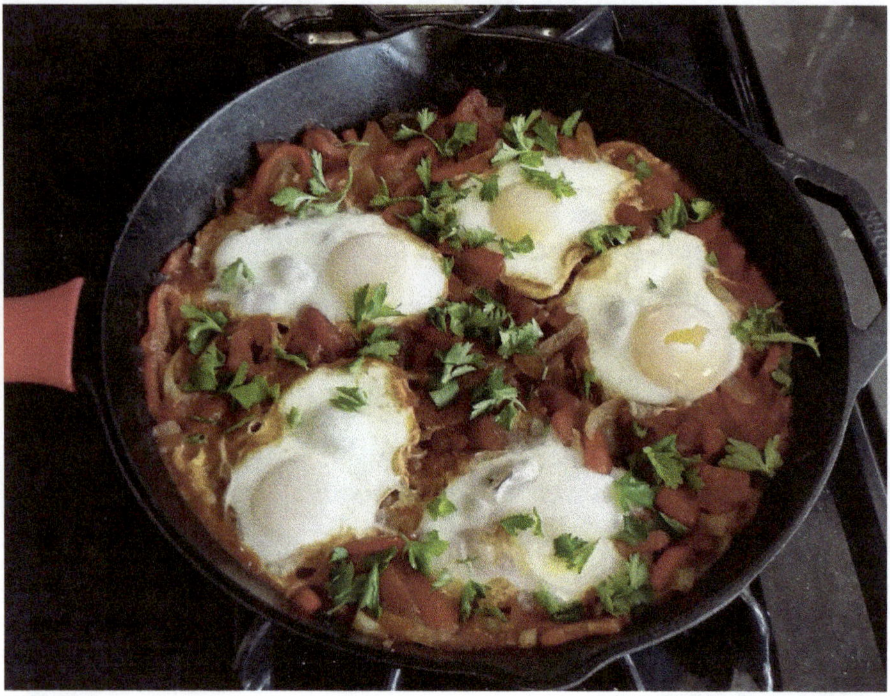

Delicious Potato Patties

Cooking Time:
20 minutes
Servings:4

Ingredients:

4 potatoes, shredded

1 onion, chopped

1 egg, beaten

¼ cup milk

2 tbsp butter

½ tsp garlic powder

Salt and black pepper to taste

3 tbsp flour

Directions:

1.Preheat air fryer to 390 F. In a bowl, add the egg, potatoes, onion, milk, butter, black pepper, flour, garlic powder, and salt and mix well to form a batter.

2.Mold the mixture into four patties. Place the patties in a greased frying basket and Air Fryer for 14-16 minutes, flipping once. Serve warm. enjoy!

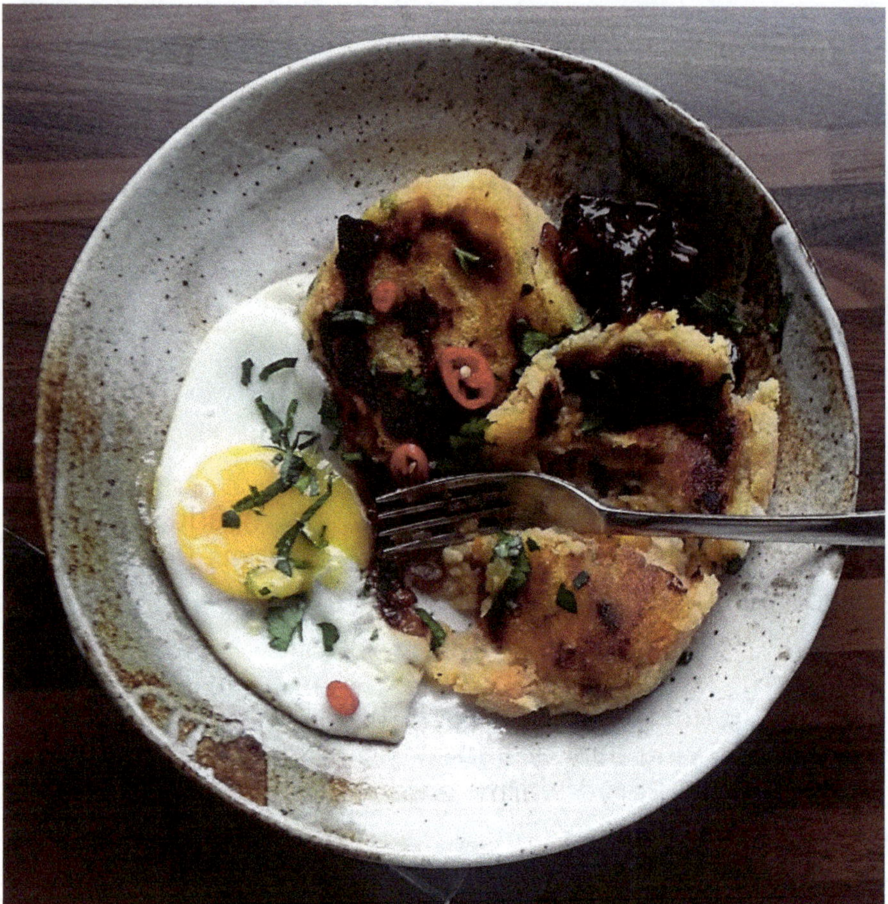

Cheesy Potatoes & Asparagus

Cooking Time:

30 minutes

Servings:5

Ingredients:

4 potatoes, cut into wedges

1 bunch asparagus, trimmed

2 tbsp olive oil

¼ cup buttermilk

¼ cup cottage cheese, crumbled

1 tbsp whole-grain mustard

Salt and black pepper to taste

Directions:

1.Preheat air fryer to 400 F. Place the potatoes in a greased frying basket and Bake for 20-22 minutes; remove and cover with foil to keep warm.

2.Drizzle asparagus with olive oil and season with salt and black pepper.

3.Bake them in the air fryer for 6-8 minutes, shaking halfway through the cooking time.

4.In a bowl, mix the cottage cheese, buttermilk, and whole-grain mustard. Arrange potatoes and asparagus on a serving platter and drizzle with the cheese sauce. Serve and enjoy!

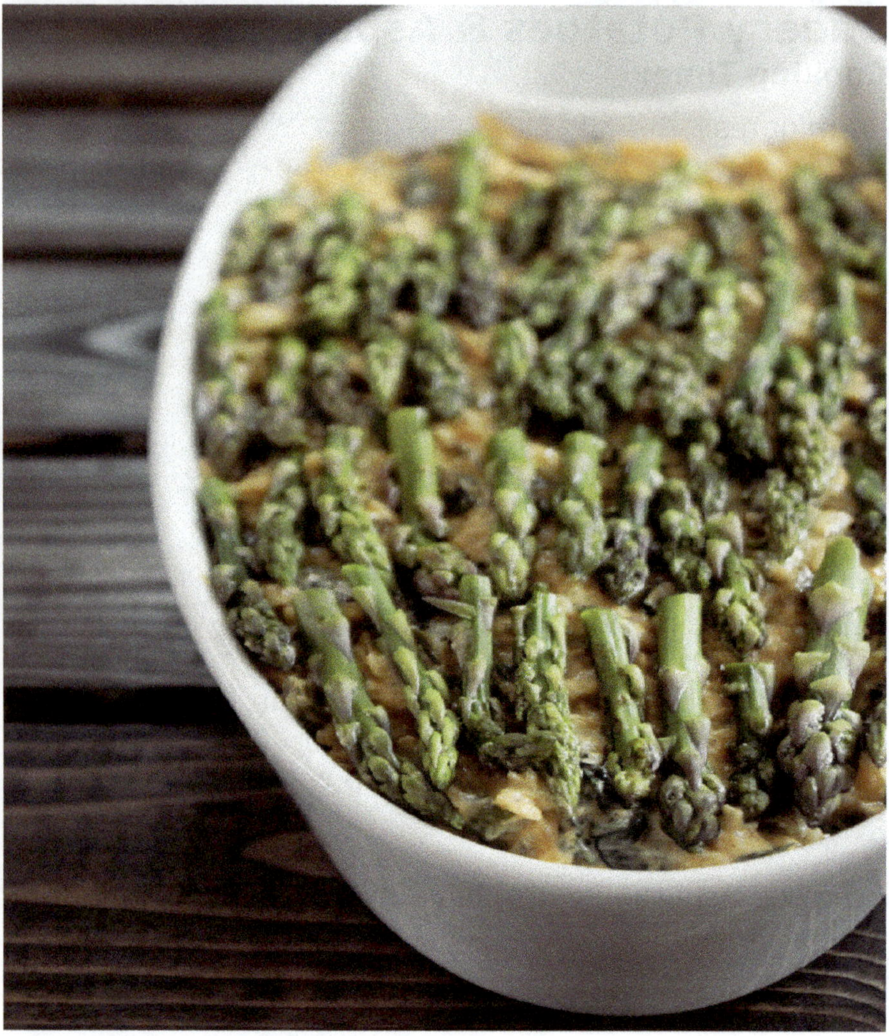

Bulgarian Red Pepper "Burek"

Cooking Time:

25 minutes

Servings:4

Ingredients:

4 red bell peppers, roasted
1 cup feta cheese, crumbled
4 eggs
1 cup breadcrumbs
4 garlic cloves, chopped
1 tomato, peeled and chopped
1 tsp fresh dill, chopped
1 tbsp fresh parsley, chopped
Salt and black pepper to taste
1 tbsp olive oil
½ cup flour 1 cup plain yogurt

DIRECTIONS

1.In a small bowl, mix the yogurt with olive oil, half of the garlic, and dill. Keep the sauce in the fridge. Preheat air fryer to 350 F.

2.In a bowl, beat 3 eggs with salt and pepper. Add in feta cheese, the remaining garlic, tomato, and parsley and mix to combine.

3.Fill the peppers with the mixture. Beat the remaining egg with salt and pepper in a bowl. Coat the peppers with flour first, then dip in the egg, and finally in the crumbs.

4.Arrange on the greased frying basket and Air Fryer for 10-12 minutes until golden brown. Serve the peppers with the yogurt sauce on the side. enjoy!

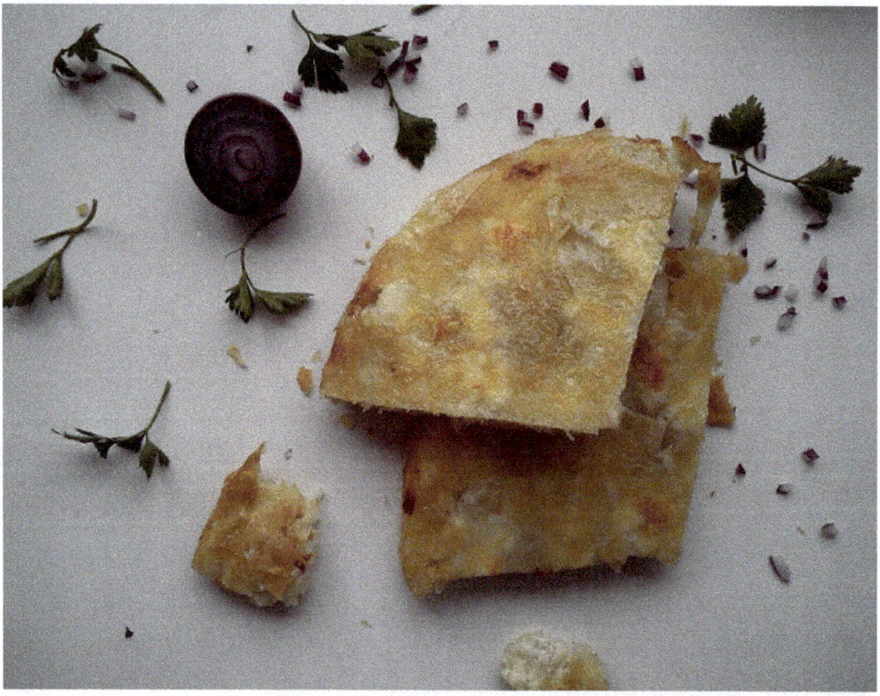

Green Pea Arancini with Tomato Sauce

Cooking Time:

60 minutes

Servings:4

Ingredients:

1cup rice, rinsed
½ green peas
1 tbsp butter
1 onion, chopped
2 garlic cloves, minced
1 egg
3 tbsp Parmesan cheese, shredded
½ cup breadcrumbs
2 tbsp olive oil
Salt and black pepper to taste
1 lb Roma tomatoes, chopped
2 tbsp fresh basil, chopped

DIRECTIONS

1.Fill a shallow saucepan with water and place over medium heat. Bring to a boil and add in the rice, salt, and pepper.

2.Cook for 20-22 minutes, stirring often. Drain rice and place in a bowl; mix in green peas.

3.Melt the butter in a skillet over medium heat and sauté onion and garlic for 3 minutes until soft. Remove the mixture to the rice bowl and add in Parmesan cheese and egg; mix well.

4.Mold the mixture into golf-size balls and roll them in breadcrumbs.

5.Place on a baking sheet and refrigerate for 1 hour. Heat the olive oil in the skillet and cook the tomatoes for 6-8 minutes, stirring occasionally until the sauce thickens.

6.Season with salt and pepper. Scatter basil on top and set aside. Preheat air fryer to 360 F. Remove the arancini from the fridge and arrange them on the greased frying basket.

7.AirFry for 14-16 minutes, shaking from time to time until nicely browned. Serve with the sauce. enjoy!

Zucchini Fries with Tabasco Dip

Cooking Time:
25 minutes
Servings:4

Ingredients:
1zucchinis, sliced
2 egg whites
½ cup seasoned breadcrumbs
2 tbsp Parmesan cheese, grated
¼ tsp garlic powder
Salt and black pepper to taste
1 cup mayonnaise
¼ cup heavy cream
1 tbsp Tabasco sauce
1 tsp lime juice

DIRECTIONS

1.Preheat air fryer to 400 F. In a bowl, beat egg whites with salt and pepper.

2.In another bowl, mix garlic powder, Parmesan cheese, and breadcrumbs.

3.Dip zucchini in the egg whites, followed by breadcrumbs. Add to the greased frying basket and Air Fryer for 14 minutes, turning once halfway through.

4.In a small bowl, mix mayonnaise, heavy cream, Tabasco sauce, and lime juice. Serve on the side of the zucchini. enjoy!

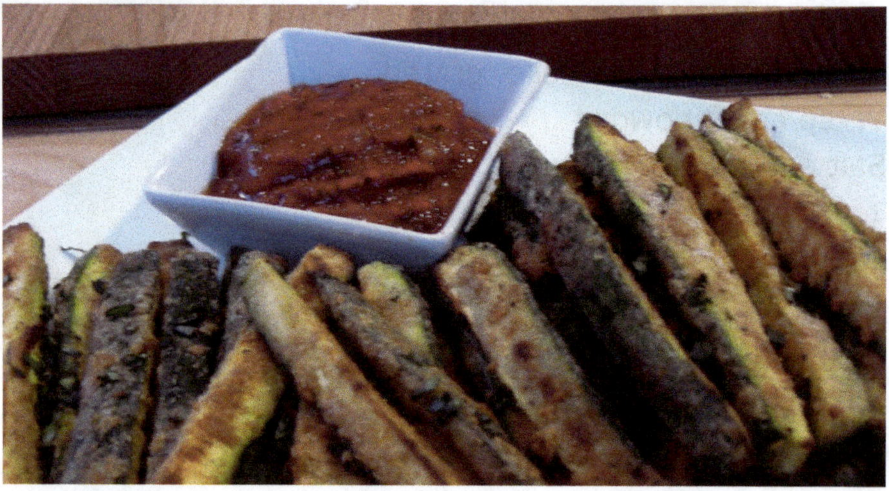

Effortless Eggplant Cheeseburger

Cooking Time:
10 minutes
Servings:4

Ingredients:
1hamburger bun
2-inch eggplant slice, cut along the round axis
1 mozzarella slice
1 red onion cut into
3 rings
1 lettuce leaf
½ tbsp tomato sauce
1 pickle, sliced

Directions:

1.Preheat air fryer to 330 F. Place the eggplant in a greased frying basket and Bake for 6 minutes, flipping once.

2.Top with the mozzarella slice and cook for 30 more seconds. Spread the tomato sauce on one half of the bun.

3.Lay the lettuce leaf on top, then lay the cheesy eggplant, onion rings, and sliced pickles. Finish with the other bun half. Serve immediately. enjoy!

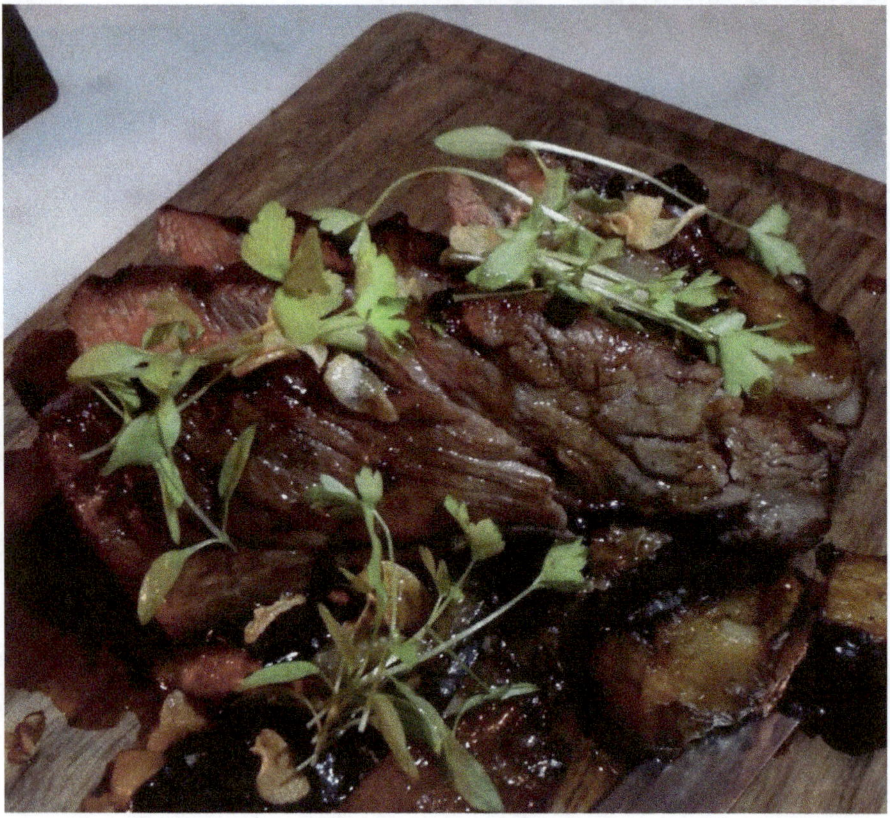

Quick Beetroot Chips

Cooking Time:
20 minutes
Servings:2

Ingredients:

1golden beetroots, thinly sliced

2 tbsp olive oil

1 tbsp yeast flakes

1 tsp Italian seasoning

Salt to taste

DIRECTIONS

1.Preheat air fryer to 360 F. In a bowl, add olive oil, beetroot slices, Italian seasoning, and yeast and mix well.

2.Dump the coated chips in the greased frying basket and Air Fryer for 12 minutes, shaking once. enjoy!

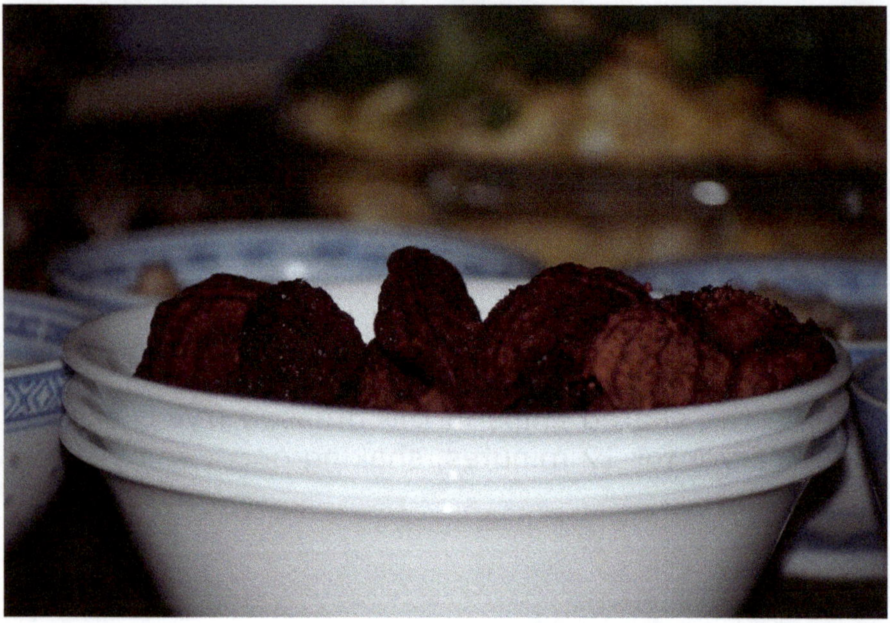

Aunt's Shallot & Carrot Bake

Cooking Time:
25 minutes
Servings:4

Ingredients:

2 tsp olive oil

2 shallots, chopped

3 carrots, sliced

Salt to taste

¼ cup yogurt

2 garlic cloves, minced

2 tbsp fresh parsley, chopped

DIRECTIONS

1.Preheat air fryer to 370 F. In a bowl, mix carrots, salt, garlic, shallots, parsley, and yogurt. Drizzle with olive oil.

2.Transfer to a greased baking dish and Bake in the air fryer for 15 minutes, shaking once. enjoy!

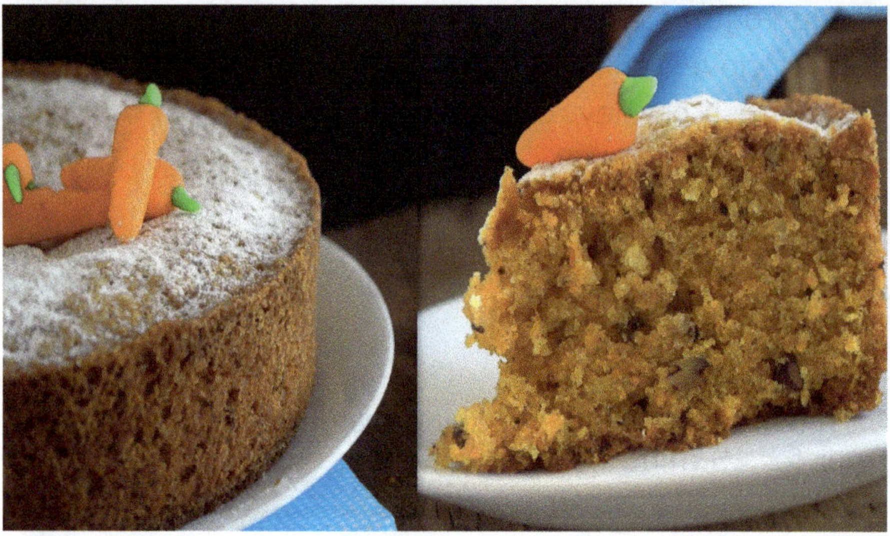

Air Fried Parmesan Cauliflower

Cooking Time:
25 minutes
Servings:4
Ingredients:

1 head of cauliflower, cut into florets

2 tbsp olive oil

4 tbsp Parmesan cheese, grated

Salt and black pepper to taste

DIRECTIONS

1.In a bowl, mix cauliflower, olive oil, salt, and black pepper.

2.Transfer to the greased frying basket and Bake for 8-10 minutes at 360 F, shaking once, until crispy. Serve sprinkled with Parmesan cheese. enjoy!

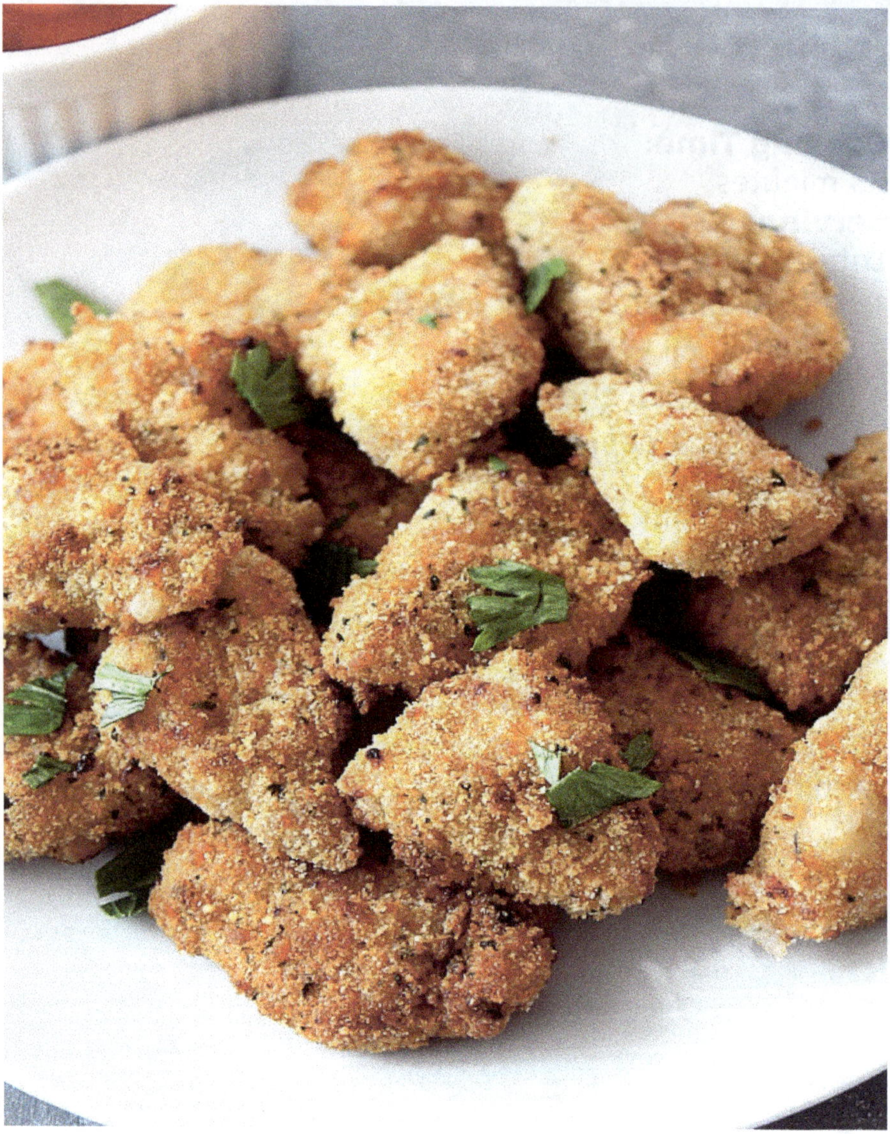

www.ingramcontent.com/pod-product-compliance
Lightning Source LLC
Chambersburg PA
CBHW050751030426
42336CB00012B/1761